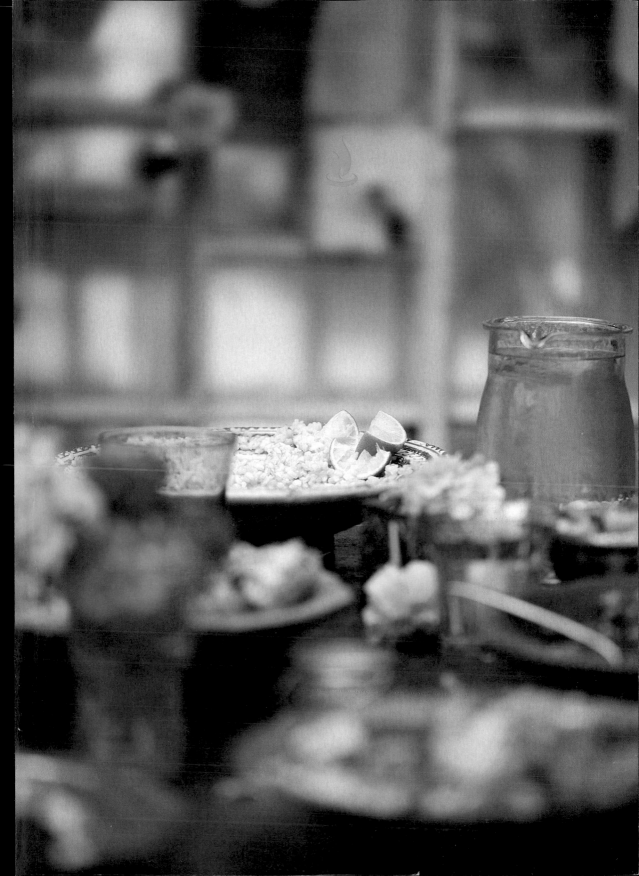

Also by Ella Mills

*Deliciously Ella: 100+ Easy, Healthy,
and Delicious Plant-Based, Gluten-Free Recipes*

*Deliciously Ella Every Day: Quick and Easy Recipes
for Gluten-Free Snacks, Packed Lunches, and Simple Meals*

Natural Feasts

100+ Healthy, Plant-Based Recipes
to Share and Enjoy with Friends and Family

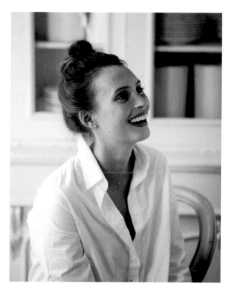

Ella Mills

SCRIBNER

New York   London   Toronto   Sydney   New Delhi

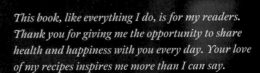

*This book, like everything I do, is for my readers.
Thank you for giving me the opportunity to share
health and happiness with you every day. Your love
of my recipes inspires me more than I can say.*

*It's also for my husband, Matthew, and our amazing
team at Deliciously Ella and the delis; without their
love and support, none of this would be possible.*

CONTENTS

Natural
Feasts

INTRODUCTION

FOREWORD

I never expected my blog, *Deliciously Ella*, to grow into the community it is now. As many of you know, my journey started back in 2011 after I was diagnosed with an illness called Postural Tachycardia Syndrome. It had a pretty devastating effect on my life, both mentally and physically. I started reading all I could find about the link between diet and lifestyle, and the way they can help manage illnesses. I was incredibly inspired by what I was learning and decided to change my life by adopting a whole-foods, plant-based diet and removing most processed foods from my meals.

Slowly but surely, I began to regain control of my symptoms. It took me about two years, but eventually I came off my medication, and I've been working on stabilizing the condition ever since. I have recurrences every now and again, but I'm now able to live the life that I want to and no longer feel held back by this chronic illness. It's been a challenging but incredibly empowering process. I never thought I'd be a businesswoman or an entrepreneur, but over the last few years my husband, Matthew, and I have spent all of our waking time creating a company in London that is passionate about natural food, the environment and social responsibility. Our passion is to change the conversation and perception around natural food.

Deliciously Ella has always served two purposes—inspiring me to learn to cook and giving me a positive outlet, both of which hugely helped me to become the person I am today. Sharing what I was learning was my way of turning a negative into a positive and it's been truly amazing to see so many people enjoy the recipes. More than anything I've wanted to use this space to show how easy it is to create beautiful, nourishing and, most important, delicious meals from simple, natural ingredients.

As the community grew, so did my following in the United States—a country I count as one of my major sources of inspiration. I spent a few months living in Venice Beach in 2014 and was incredibly energized by the food scene there. It's influenced so much of what Matt and I have done so far—with our delis in London, with the cookbooks and the app—and I'm really excited to start spending more time in the US and to get to know you all!

INTRODUCTION

Over the last few years healthy eating has really grown in popularity, which has been wonderful to watch! It's given me such a thrill to see people realize how good they feel when they eat foods that nourish their bodies. The best part of it all, though, is that everyone's started to see how incredibly delicious healthy living can be. The stereotype that it's all about lettuce and cucumber is vanishing and is being replaced with dreamy visions of blueberry pancake stacks with caramelized banana bites and crunchy cacao and almond butter, bowls of creamy sweet potato noodles with satay sauce, mango and mushroom ceviche and chocolate orange tart.

So many of my readers say that they love eating whole foods and incorporating plant-based meals into their routine . . . but that their husbands, wives, children, friends and colleagues are more skeptical and, as a result, they're not particularly open-minded about trying new, veggie-laden dishes. Lots of people also struggle to know what to cook and how to put menus together when they're entertaining, especially when they're new to this way of eating. When I first started eating a plant-based diet, I found it hard to know which dishes would complement each other best. I got it really wrong a few times with my friends and I'm pretty sure they left the table thinking I was a bit mad! The good news is that this book is designed to solve both these issues.

Each chapter is focused on delicious meals. I've got your mornings covered with brunches and breakfasts, followed by lighter meals that work well on the go; big healthy feasts and celebration menus; essential side dishes, party staples and, of course, everyone's favorite—desserts. I've also given meal suggestions that cater to your every sociable need: think brunch for the girls, or a grab-and-go breakfast, pantry saviors, delights for your desk, cold-weather comforters, Mexican fiestas and even dishes—such as a knockout Sunday lunch—designed to impress the skeptics in your life! So once you've worked your way through the book you'll feel inspired, knowing exactly how to put Deliciously Ella–style meals together in a way that persuades your friends and family to try some healthy versions of their favorites. Plus, you'll get to cook more than one hundred delicious new recipes. We'll be making so many lovely things, from peanut butter and jelly cake to quesadillas stuffed with garlicky beans, cashew sour cream, salsa and guacamole; almond butter rocky roads; pea, zucchini and coconut risotto; chickpea chili with baked sweet potatoes; and chocolate peanut butter pie! Get ready: this is a seriously tasty book.

We'll start with my favorite breakfast and brunch recipes: think on-the-go menus with crumbly blueberry squares, roasted almond butter bars and honey and lemon breakfast bars. Or awesome savory brunches with stacks of sweet potato rösti piled high with maple and rosemary butter beans and spread with a thick layer of herby guacamole. We're also having toasted buckwheat and coconut granola with zesty mango and pineapple bowls and passion fruit yogurt, as well as baked garlicky tomatoes, scrambled turmeric and red pepper tofu and thyme fried mushrooms. There's a great range of options, from easy dishes you can throw together to help rushed mornings when you're time poor, to fancy brunches to share on lazy weekends.

We'll then go through some fantastic lighter recipes that work well for quick weekday suppers, as well as portable lunches. We'll look at fresh bites like mango and mushroom ceviche and sushi rolls filled with cauliflower rice, sesame and avocado; after-work catch-up menus of spiced potato cakes

with garlicky tomato sauce and green beans; and perfect picnics with charred coconut corn and vibrant salads filled with mango, pepper, cucumber and a peanut dressing. This chapter is full of my go-to meals, quick and easy, but still so delicious! The chile and ginger pho, sesame slaw, pistachio and apricot quinoa and sesame and maple summer rolls are real favorites here. I make these for Matt and me during the week when we're at home, or when I have a couple of girlfriends coming over for weekday supper.

The next chapter is all about hearty feasts and celebrations. These are the meals I make when I have lots of friends and family over, or want to impress someone! I promise all these dishes and menus will convince any skeptic that eating well can be pretty amazing. There's a great selection of ideas in here, from Mexican-themed feasts, to curries with homemade lime pickle, to warming meals of

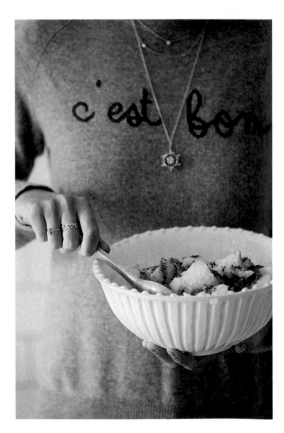

tomato and eggplant bake served alongside bowls of spinach with mustard seeds. We then cover everything from garden parties filled with charred cauliflower steaks on a bed of chile quinoa and sun-dried tomato and butter bean hummus, to comforting bowls of three-bean stew with mango salsa, to simple, inexpensive suppers of spiced chickpea chili stuffed into baked sweet potatoes. There's really something for everyone.

After this we move toward side dishes. This is probably my favorite chapter of the book as there's such a wide range of ingredients, flavors and textures here. I absolutely love using these as traditional sides, but it's also fun to make a few of these recipes and throw them into a bowl together to make a full meal. It always looks beautiful and tastes sensational. I have so many much-loved recipes in this chapter, but the baked plantains with a sweet chile sauce, the smashed potatoes with turmeric and mustard seeds, the miso and sesame glazed eggplants and the spicy baked avocado fries with their lime, cashew and cilantro dip are all absolute winners . . . and you all should try them. I have a feeling that they'll become staples in your diet too. There's a good mix of impressive and simple dishes in this chapter, so there should be something to suit every taste bud and every occasion. The other great thing about the recipes in this chapter is that you can mix and match them with just about anything, so if you're not ready to go fully Deliciously Ella, then just add these to your existing go-to meals. That way you can experiment with new ingredients without it all feeling too new and overwhelming. If you're a meat eater, then these are great ways to incorporate a bit more plant-based goodness into your diet too, and hopefully they'll get you excited about how good veggies can taste.

To make things more fun I've dedicated a whole chapter to parties; we've got nibbles, cocktails and mocktails and even birthday teas! You'll be able to serve a lovely array of little bites, from charred Padrón peppers with chipotle cream to bowls of smoky baked tortilla chips with babaganoush,

eggplant rolls with a minty coconut tzatziki and mini baked potatoes with cashew sour cream and chives, as well as mini socca pizza bites. To accompany them there's a list of mocktails and cocktails, so you and your friends can sip on sparkling pineapple and cayenne drinks, or watermelon and cucumber coolers as you catch up. And to end the chapter we've got a beautiful afternoon tea with iced ginger muffins, a banana and raisin cake and simple cucumber and lemon butter bean hummus open sandwiches, as well as a birthday tea with peanut butter and honey oat bars, blueberry scones with vanilla coconut cream and a triple-layered celebration cake. I think this chapter will really show your friends and family that healthy eating is accessible, delicious and sociable—it's absolutely not about sitting on your own at home every night meditating and eating kale salad! These dishes are amazing if you want to do a big dinner party, too, as they mean you can keep it delicious but with a healthy twist from start to finish!

To end the book we'll go through all the best sweet ways to finish a meal. I know how much my readers love sweets and there are some real winners in this chapter, which I'm sure you'll all really enjoying making, eating and sharing (if there's any left by the time your friends arrive!). We've got beautiful desserts like pistachio and orange truffles, watermelon and mint granita, pan-fried cardamom and honey apples and berries with creamy chocolate sauce and crushed nuts, which work so well as lighter options at the end of a meal. There are also lots of amazing snacks, from salted maca and tahini fudge, to orange and cardamom cookies and my personal favorite—quinoa, hazelnut and cacao bars—that work really well on the go. Then, if you're looking for something heartier and more indulgent, there are some wonders for you near the end of the chapter as we move toward chocolate peanut butter pie, glazed orange polenta cake and even a sticky toffee pudding. There's so much here for everyone, and I'm sure these will all go over really well with your friends and family.

Hopefully the recipes, ideas and menus that

you'll see throughout the book will inspire you to get cooking, so that you can enjoy amazing food with the people you love. Of course, you don't have to use the book in this way; I pull out single recipes and make them on their own all the time, as they're all so great and obviously you won't necessarily want to make a full three-course meal every night! I've just put them together to help you work out what goes well with what, so that you feel confident in the kitchen.

HOW TO MAKE HEALTHY EATING APPROACHABLE FOR EVERYONE

While I am on the subject of sharing food with others, including those who might be more skeptical about eating plant-based food, the other point I'd like to highlight is that eating well is not about labels, guilt or enforcing a certain way of eating on yourself or anyone else. It's so important to remember this, especially when you're introducing your friends and family to this kind of food, as you don't want them to feel too overwhelmed and daunted by the concept.

The way we eat is so personal to us, and we are all different. We have different bodies, different medical histories, different genes, different lifestyles and different tastes. I do believe that everyone is better off—both physically and mentally—with a diet full of fruit, veg, nuts, seeds, beans, legumes, healthy grains, and less refined sugar and processed food . . . but, after that, you have to make your own decisions, and it's OK if these are different from the choices made by your friends and family. Only you know what's practical, enjoyable and sustainable for your lifestyle and, as with anything in life, the way you eat doesn't fall into a one-size-fits-all bucket.

Healthy eating is about finding a way of eating that makes you happy. It's about meals that make you feel your best—that might mean a crumbly blueberry square for breakfast, a lemony potato and butter bean salad for lunch . . . and then a pizza with wine for dinner with friends—and that's totally OK. It's your body and your life. Yes, I want to encourage

everyone to show their bodies some love and take good care of them, but I never ever want anyone to feel guilty because they're not eating "perfectly" all the time. Plus, there is no such thing as perfect—perfect is simply finding a balance that is right for you, whatever that is.

This book is all about natural, plant-based food and the recipes are all vegetarian and wheat-free, but there are no labels on any of it. It's simply about delicious food that's designed to help you feel good, and you can adapt any of it. As you read this book, please don't feel you have to put yourself firmly into any dietary "category." Putting yourself in a certain box with a specific label can be quite restrictive. You just shouldn't feel that you're not healthy if you're not specifically raw, plant-based, Paleo, grain-free, gluten-free, wheat-free or any of the rest of it. You can absolutely be a bit of everything, you just have to be honest with yourself and work out what makes you feel best . . . and that might be a happy mix of everything. Of course it can also mean following a certain concept, but please don't feel as though it's wrong if you don't. Likewise, you shouldn't expect anyone else you know and love to categorize themselves either. Don't forget that healthy eating should never be prescriptive or restricting!

The other thing to note is that we also all want to commit to healthy eating to different extents and that's great. I eat the way I do because I love it, but also because it's the only way that I'm able to manage my illness. I want to—and have to—eat nourishing food all the time. Just because I eat this way every day, though, doesn't mean you should feel bad if you don't. Similarly, you shouldn't inflict guilt on anyone else if they're not ready to eat healthily all day long either, just focus on encouraging them to add more natural foods to their diet and celebrate the small steps and changes that they're making rather than focusing on the other things you feel they could be doing. We all respond so much better to positivity than negativity.

So please remember that when you're

introducing friends and family to this food, it's important to let them know that it's totally OK to be a flexible healthy eater and that—just because you live with someone or spend a lot of time together—it doesn't mean you have to eat in exactly the same way. Everyone has to start somewhere, at some point, and it's much better to introduce healthy living to your own or someone else's life in a sustainable way over time than it is to do it all at once . . . and then quit three days later because you/they hate living on kale salads.

Find a balance that works for you and the people around you, incorporate whole ingredients and nourishing foods whenever you can and—most important—please don't beat yourself up or make anyone else feel bad for eating something that isn't super healthy . . . because life is much too short for that!

TOP TIPS FOR ENCOURAGING FRIENDS AND FAMILY TO GET HEALTHIER

1 FOCUS ON FAMILIAR FOOD
If you're having a real skeptic for dinner, or trying to get an unconvinced family member to try a healthier meal, then always cook something that looks and feels familiar to them. Choose a classic dish that has a healthy spin on it. Something like quesadillas and cashew sour cream and guacamole. This is a perfect meal, as your guests are never going to look at it and think, "What is that, it looks terrifyingly healthy!" and decide they don't like it before they try it, plus it's really satisfying and hearty, which means everyone will go home full. So remember to go easy on everyone, don't leap straight to raw food, or anything too unfamiliar and scary looking!

2 DEMONSTRATE, DON'T PREACH
No one likes to be preached at or made to feel guilty about anything in life, especially the way they eat, as it's often attached to a lot of emotions and possibly deep-rooted insecurities. Don't talk about meals as being "good" or "bad" healthwise: there's no point categorizing anything to inflict guilt. Instead just demonstrate how delicious healthy

food is. Make your friends amazing, nourishing meals and encourage them to try them, but without telling them why it's so much better than what they normally eat. Simply cook and share natural goodness; that's exactly how I got all my friends and family involved. If you do want to inspire them with the benefits of healthy eating, then let them know how good you've been feeling since you started incorporating more whole foods into your diet, and how much your own energy levels—and everything else—have improved . . . but just don't go on about it too much!

3 IT'S OK TO ADAPT ALL THE RECIPES
As I said earlier, healthy eating isn't about labeling yourself or forcing yourself to do something you don't enjoy. If you're new to healthy eating, or trying to get friends and family involved, don't be afraid to adapt any of my recipes to make them more accessible for your audience. If adding chicken,

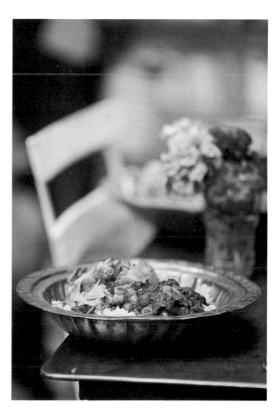

fish, cheese or eggs makes the people you love more likely to try something new, then add them in by all means; if it makes them more receptive and allows them to enjoy the meal more, then that's a great thing. It also means their plate will look more familiar, which I find is the best approach.

4 DON'T CHANGE EVERYTHING AT ONCE

You don't have to overhaul your diet overnight. There's no rush or deadline for changing your lifestyle. It's about finding an enjoyable, sustainable way of life that makes you happy and it really doesn't matter how long it takes to get there! Start by focusing on positives and adding goodness in, rather than taking everything away. Add in new veggie dishes throughout the week, but don't feel you have to remove the old favorites at the same time; just let the two coexist for a while as you get used to new ways of eating and cooking. Allow yourself and the people around you however long you and they need to start loving the new ingredients, textures and tastes. Most important, never criticize yourself if you don't enjoy something! You don't have to love all fruit and veg; even I don't enjoy them all—you'll never find me eating iceberg lettuce or green peppers for example—but that's OK, there are so many other lovely ingredients out there to experiment with instead.

5 DON'T BE TOO STRICT ON YOURSELF OR ANYONE ELSE

It's so important to remember that no one is perfect, and there's no point in striving for perfection, as the concept simply doesn't exist. This is relevant to everything in life really, but I believe it's especially important to remember when thinking about food. When it comes to what we eat and how we eat, we just have to do what makes us feel happiest and never forget that this will be different for everyone. Food is such an important part of life and you don't want to feel stressed every time you sit down for a meal, which takes away all the fun from something you should really look forward to and savor. So find a balance that you enjoy and, if you lapse from your

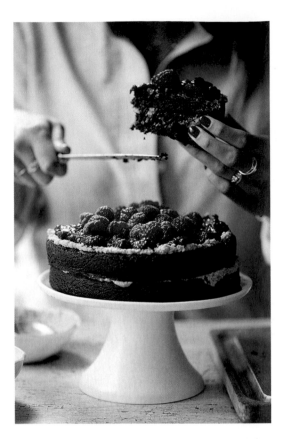

healthy-eating plan, never beat yourself up, just find a positive way to get back into it; we're all only human after all! Every change in life also takes time to become a habit, so don't expect yourself to wake up craving quinoa on day one; sadly it's unlikely to happen. Just be OK with that, accept where you are right now and, crucially, don't judge what you are craving: embrace it . . . and then try to incorporate a healthy something on the side!

6 MAKE THE MEAL BEAUTIFUL

Concentrate on making the food you serve look really appetizing. It may sound like a bit of a waste of time, but it's not. We eat with our eyes first, so a dish needs to look tempting, especially if you're trying to get someone new excited about it. If you and your guests think it looks amazing, you'll all be much more open-minded and ready for it to taste amazing, too. This has been one of the most important things for me as Deliciously Ella, especially on the blog and Instagram. So many readers have said that they tried something they thought they wouldn't like because it looked great, and they ended up loving it! It doesn't take long to enhance the appearance of something. You just need to put it in a clean, beautiful serving dish (rather than serving it in what you cooked it in) and then add a little color and texture with dressings, herb sprinklings and toppings such as toasted nuts and pomegranates.

7 KEEP THE INGREDIENTS A SECRET

This may sound a bit strange, but I find it really helps people be more objective if they don't know there's a certain ingredient in a dish. Lots of us think we hate a particular taste or texture, but if we try it in a new context, we often end up loving it. I've had so many friends say, "Oh I hate dates," but then they love my crunchy almond butter rocky roads and eat three of them, or they say they hate cilantro but adore the spiced potato cakes. Especially if it's just one of many ingredients, it's worth keeping it a secret so that they try it with an open mind . . . and I think you'll both be surprised by the result! (Obviously, make sure you know they are not allergic to it first.) If it is a main ingredient, and therefore not disguisable, then I always highlight the fact that it's been cooked in a totally different way and is being served with new flavors, to demonstrate that it's very different from how they may have had it before, and this often works too. Just do your best to encourage your friends and family to try things with an open mind and you may end up with a few new converts!

I hope my experiences, and the tips I've learned for convincing friends and family to try new things, are helpful to you all. Now, let's get cooking!

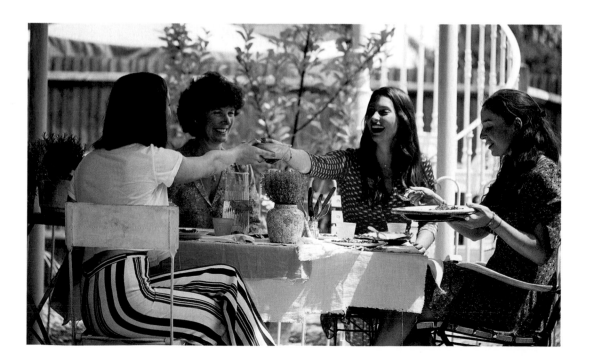

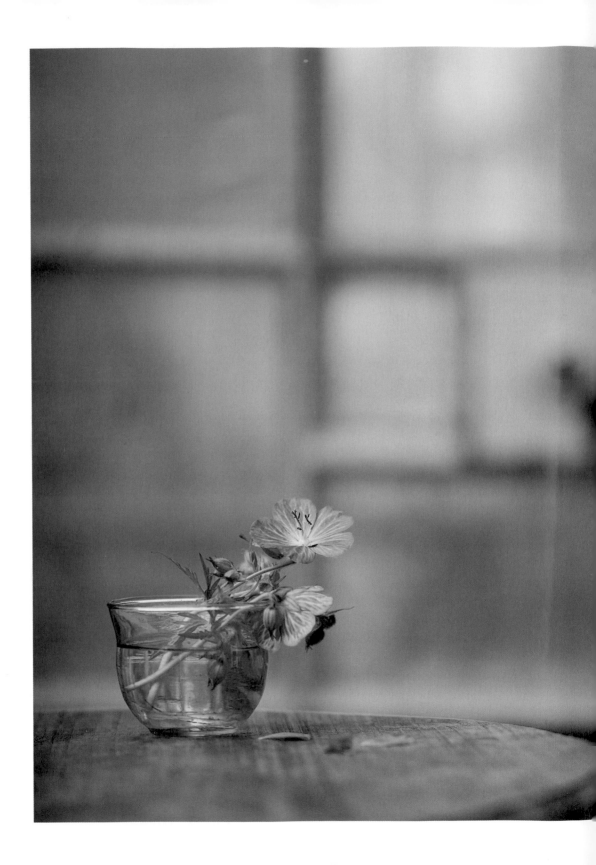

MORNINGS

BREAKFASTS & BRUNCHES TO MAKE EVERY DAY DELICIOUS

MORNINGS

*I'm a big breakfast person. I really believe that it's the most important
meal of the day, and it tends to be the one I'm most excited about.
Some days I'm really busy so I'll grab a Honey & Lemon Breakfast
Bar and a Crumbly Blueberry Square to eat on the go as I run out of
the door. Other days I have time to throw together a Zesty Mango &
Pineapple Bowl with Passion Fruit Yogurt and a sprinkling of Toasted
Buckwheat & Coconut Granola for Matt and myself, and we can spend
a few minutes savoring the flavors before the day starts. On weekends
I like to invite friends over for long, leisurely brunches and really
take my time over the meal, so you'll find me feasting on a Blueberry
Pancake Stack with Caramelized Banana Bites and dollops
of homemade Crunchy Cacao & Almond Butter.*

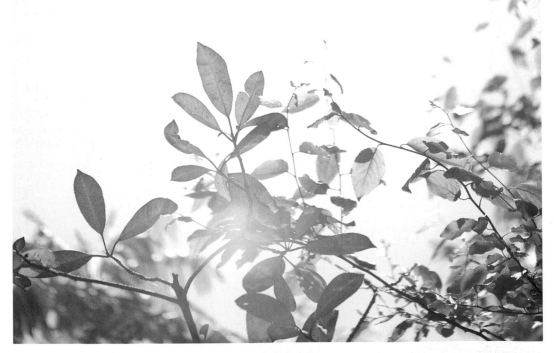

MENUS

GRAB & GO
Honey & Lemon Breakfast Bars
Crumbly Blueberry Squares
Roasted Almond Butter Bars

US TIME
Matt's Berry & Orange Smoothie
Toasted Buckwheat & Coconut Granola
Zesty Mango & Pineapple Bowls with Passion Fruit Yogurt

SWEET BRUNCH
Blueberry Pancake Stack
Caramelized Banana Bites
Crunchy Cacao & Almond Butter

THE NEW FULL ENGLISH
Scrambled Turmeric & Red Pepper Tofu
Thyme Fried Mushrooms
Garlicky Baked Tomatoes

SAVORY BRUNCH
Sweet Potato Rösti
Maple & Rosemary Butter Beans
Herby Guacamole

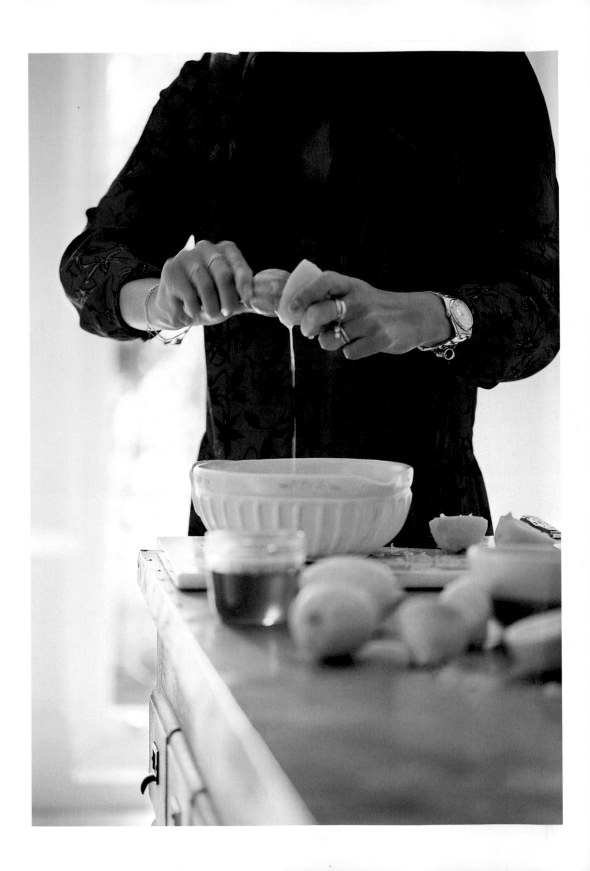

HONEY & LEMON BREAKFAST BARS

These are easy to carry around, full of flavor and simple to make. They also freeze very well, so you can make a big batch and they'll last you a long time. If you like a sweet snack in the afternoon, too, take an extra bar with you to enjoy later in the day.

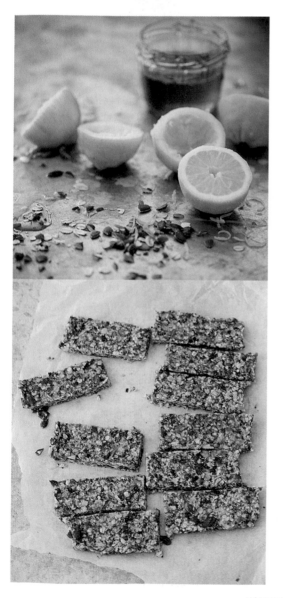

Makes 8

1 tablespoon coconut oil

3 tablespoons honey

juice and finely grated zest of 1 unwaxed lemon

1 tablespoon tahini

½ cup pumpkin seeds

6 medjool dates, pitted

1 cup plus 6 tablespoons rolled oats

2 tablespoons chia seeds

pinch of salt

Melt the coconut oil, honey, lemon juice and tahini together in a pan over a gentle heat.

Put the pumpkin seeds into a food processor and pulse a few times until they are roughly chopped. Tip into a large mixing bowl. Put the dates in the food processor and blend until a sticky paste forms. Add this to the pumpkin seeds with all the other ingredients, including the contents of the pan (and not forgetting the lemon zest). Mix thoroughly until everything is evenly coated.

Line a rimmed baking sheet with parchment paper, spoon in the mixture and press it down evenly.

Place in the fridge for about 2 hours to set. Cut into 8 squares or slices before serving.

CRUMBLY BLUEBERRY SQUARES

*I make a big batch of these every week or two, so I have great speedy options to grab
when I'm running out of the house to start the day. That makes my mornings so much
simpler . . . and way more delicious.*

Makes 16

FOR THE BASE

a little coconut oil, for the pan

4⅔ cups rolled oats

scant ½ cup brown rice milk, or other
  plant-based milk

5 tablespoons maple syrup

½ teaspoon ground cinnamon

FOR THE FILLING

2 cups blueberries

2 tablespoons maple syrup

6 medjool dates, pitted and
  roughly chopped

2 teaspoons arrowroot powder

FOR THE TOPPING

¼ cup coconut oil

2 tablespoons honey

1 teaspoon ground cinnamon

½ teaspoon ground ginger

2½ cups rolled oats

Preheat the oven to 350°F. Use the coconut oil to oil an 8-inch square brownie pan.

Start by making the base. Place all the ingredients into a food processor and pulse-blend a few times, until everything is mixed but not totally smooth. Press the mixture into the prepared pan, packing it as tightly as you can. Pop it in the oven for 15 minutes, then take out and set aside to cool.

Next make the filling. Simply place all the ingredients except the arrowroot into a saucepan with a scant ¼ cup water and cook over medium heat for about 10 minutes until the blueberries have all burst and it's starting to resemble a compote. Stir in the arrowroot and 2 more teaspoons water to help it thicken. Set aside to cool.

Meanwhile, make the topping. Melt the coconut oil, honey and spices together in a saucepan, then stir in the oats.

Pour the berry filling onto the base and spread it out evenly, then tumble over the oaty topping, pressing down lightly so that it is compact and completely covers the filling. Return it to the oven for 25–30 minutes, until the top is golden. Let cool in the pan before cutting into 16 portions.

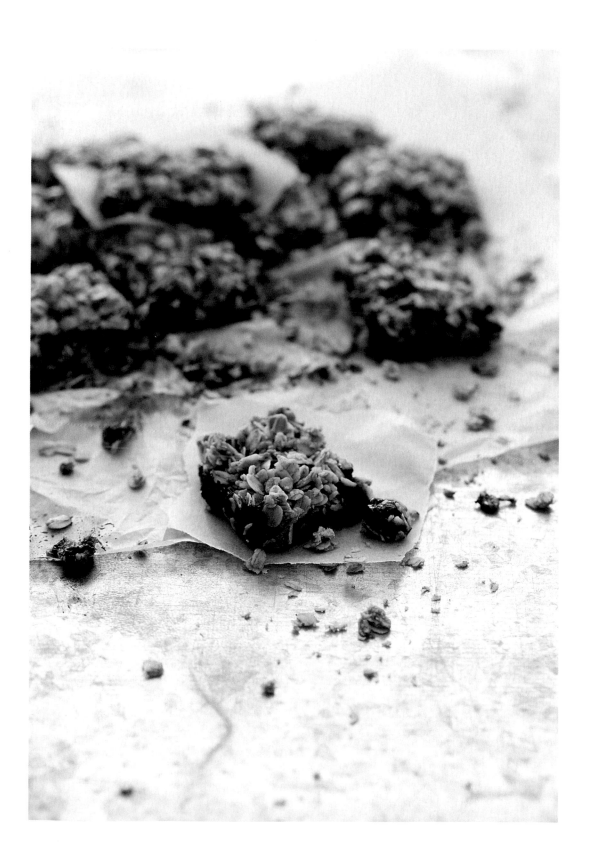

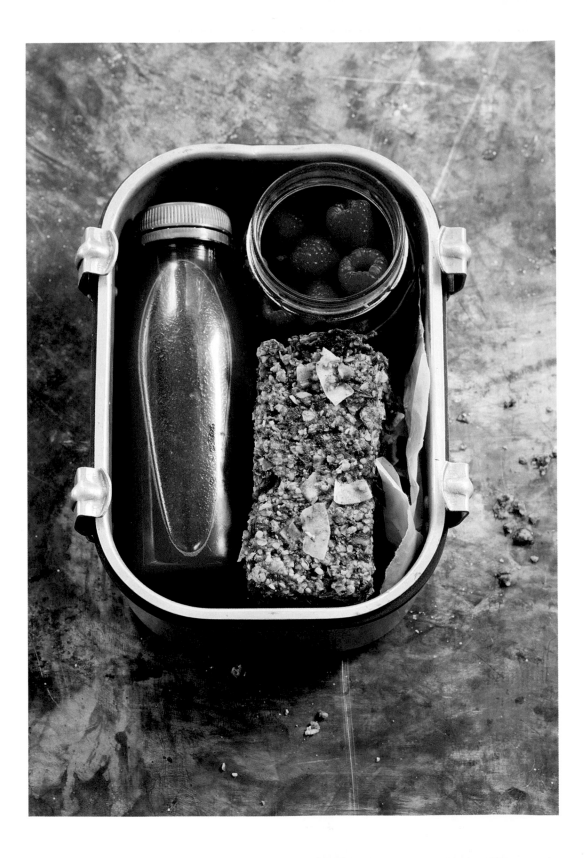

ROASTED ALMOND BUTTER BARS

An ideal option for busy mornings, wonderfully chewy with little bites of juicy raisins, coconut chips and hemp seeds. I use dates and apple purée to sweeten these, so they're not sickly sweet, making them a great way to start your day!

Makes 10–12

2 tablespoons coconut oil, plus more
    for the pan
2 tablespoons chia seeds
12 medjool dates, pitted
2½ cups rolled oats
5 tablespoons **apple purée** (see below)
2 teaspoons ground cinnamon
4 tablespoons hulled hemp seeds
3 tablespoons roasted almond butter
½ cup unsweetened coconut chips
⅓ cup raisins
pinch of salt

Preheat the oven to 400°F. Use some coconut oil to oil an 11 x 7-inch baking pan.

Put the chia in a glass with ½ cup water. Let this sit for 20 minutes until the seeds expand and form a gel.

Put the dates and the 2 tablespoons coconut oil into a food processor and whizz.

Mix all the other ingredients, including the chia gel, in a bowl, then stir in the dates until everything is evenly blended.

Press into the prepared pan and bake for about 20 minutes, or until golden brown.

CLEVER COOKING

Apple purée is a great way to sweeten lots of recipes without adding refined sugar. Simply peel and core red apples and chop them into bite-size pieces. Place in a large saucepan with ¾ inch water. Simmer for 40 minutes, or until very soft, then blend until smooth. Store in the fridge for up to 5 days, or freeze in portions.

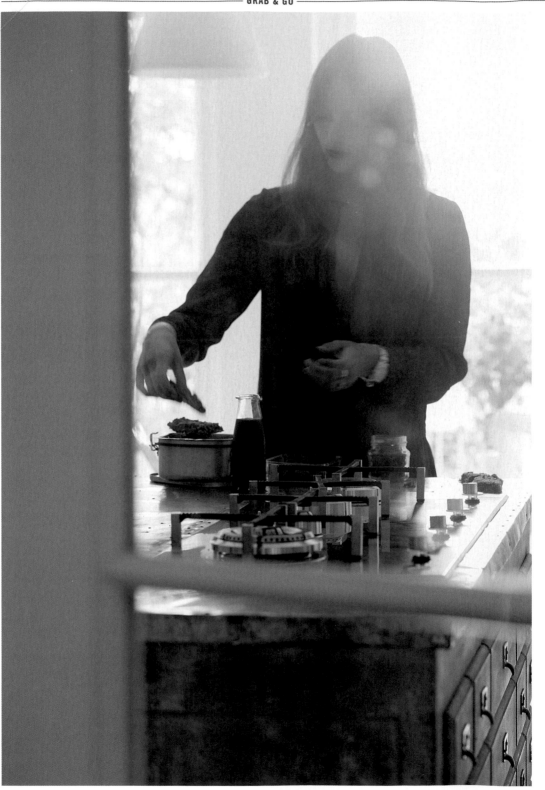

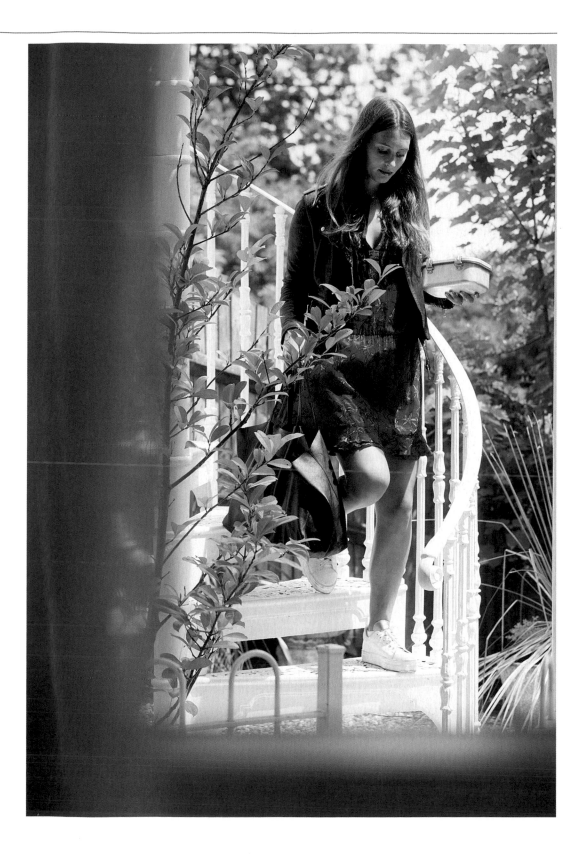

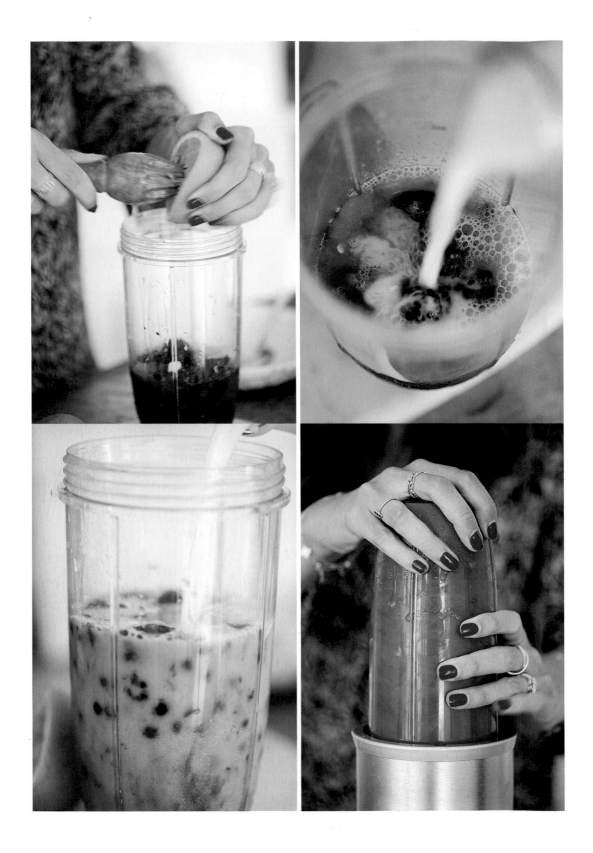

MATT'S BERRY & ORANGE SMOOTHIE

I've made this smoothie for Matt pretty much every morning for the last year! He's totally obsessed with it, and luckily for me it's easy to throw together. The frozen berries give it a lovely thick texture, while the orange and honey add great sweetness to every sip. It's a great accompaniment to Zesty Mango & Pineapple Bowls sprinkled with crunchy granola (pages 30 and 29).

Makes 1 large glass

NUT-FREE

2 oranges

¾ cup frozen mixed berries

scant ½ cup brown rice milk, or other
    plant-based milk

½ teaspoon honey (optional)

Cut the oranges in half and use a citrus squeezer to juice them into a blender.

Tip all the other ingredients into the blender, and blend until smooth.

SUPER SPEEDY

10 minutes

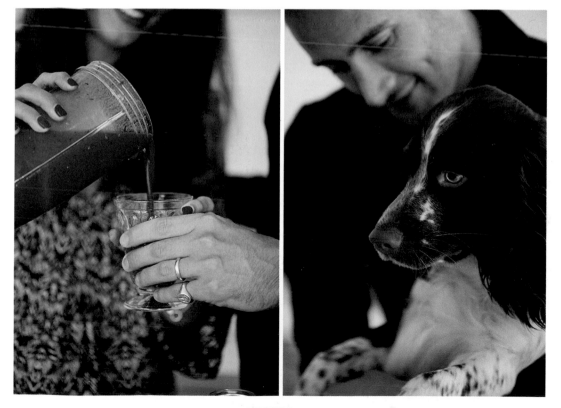

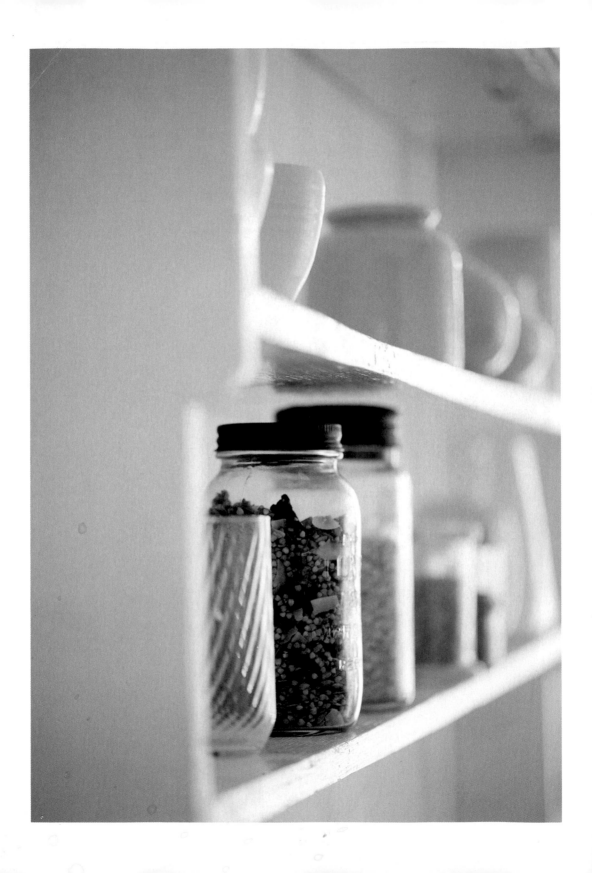

TOASTED BUCKWHEAT & COCONUT GRANOLA

I'm a complete granola addict; it's one of my favorite breakfasts, snacks and sweet treats. For me the best thing about munching on a handful of granola is the crunchy texture, which is just so incredibly satisfying. Using buckwheat groats instead of oats makes each bite especially crunchy, which is why I love this recipe so much. I toss the buckwheat in coconut oil, honey, ginger, cinnamon and vanilla, then bake it all together until my kitchen smells divine and my tummy starts rumbling!

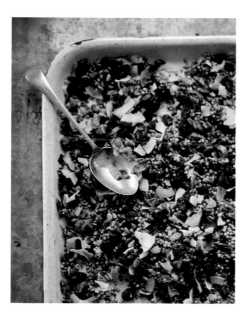

Makes 1 quart jar

1¾ cups buckwheat groats
1 cup unsweetened coconut chips
6 tablespoons sunflower seeds
¾ cup pumpkin seeds
pinch of salt
3 tablespoons coconut oil
1 tablespoon ground cinnamon
5 teaspoons ground ginger
2 teaspoons vanilla powder
3 tablespoons honey
4–6 tablespoons dried cranberries, preferably
    unsweetened (optional)
2–4 tablespoons raisins (optional)

Preheat the oven to 400°F.

Mix the buckwheat, coconut chips and seeds in a bowl with the salt.

Warm the coconut oil, cinnamon, ginger, vanilla and honey in a pan, heating gently until everything is mixed and the coconut oil has melted. Pour into the buckwheat bowl and mix everything together. Spread out evenly on a rimmed baking sheet.

Bake for 15 minutes, then give it a good stir.

Bake for another 10 minutes, stirring it halfway through.

Let it cool, then, once at room temperature, stir in any dried fruit you want and store in an airtight container. It will last in there for a couple of weeks.

ZESTY MANGO & PINEAPPLE BOWLS
WITH PASSION FRUIT YOGURT

The sweet passion fruit yogurt here tastes amazing with the mix of mango, pineapple, lime juice, maple syrup and coconut, especially when you then sprinkle granola on top. This looks amazing presented in individual glass jars with the granola topping; the layers really stand out and your friends and family will absolutely love them!

Serves 6

1 mango
½ pineapple
3 tablespoons maple syrup
¼ cup coconut chips
finely grated zest and juice of
    2 unwaxed limes
1¾ cups coconut yogurt
3 passion fruits
1¾ cups granola, plus more to serve
    (page 29 for homemade)

Start by peeling the mango and pineapple and roughly chopping them into little pieces.

In a large mixing bowl, mix the mango, pineapple, maple syrup, coconut chips and lime zest and juice. Set aside to give time for the flavors to mingle.

In a high-powered blender, whizz together the yogurt and the flesh of the passion fruits until smooth, then put the mixture in the fridge to chill.

Line up 6 jars, glasses or bowls and divide the yogurt among them, then spoon a layer of the fruit salad mix into each. Chill until you want to serve, then take them out of the fridge and sprinkle with granola.

CLEVER COOKING
Don't add the granola too far in advance or it will become soggy.

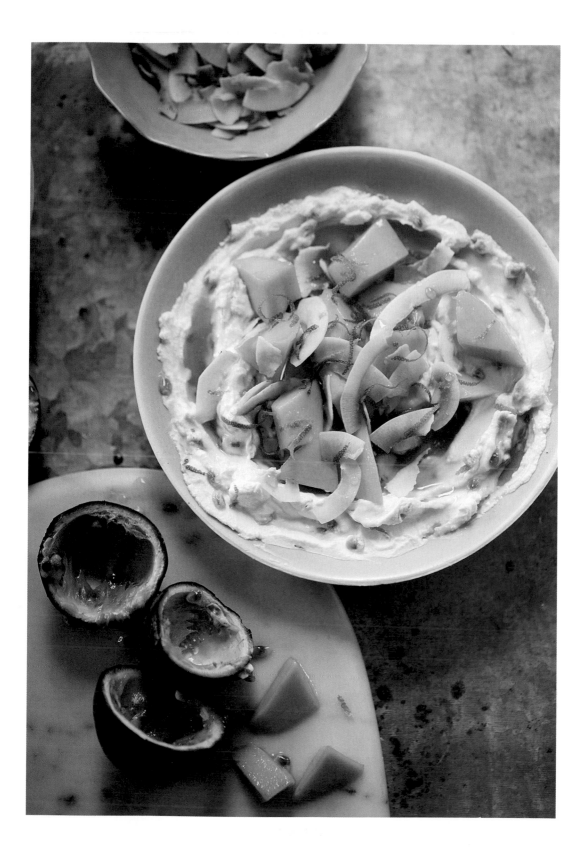

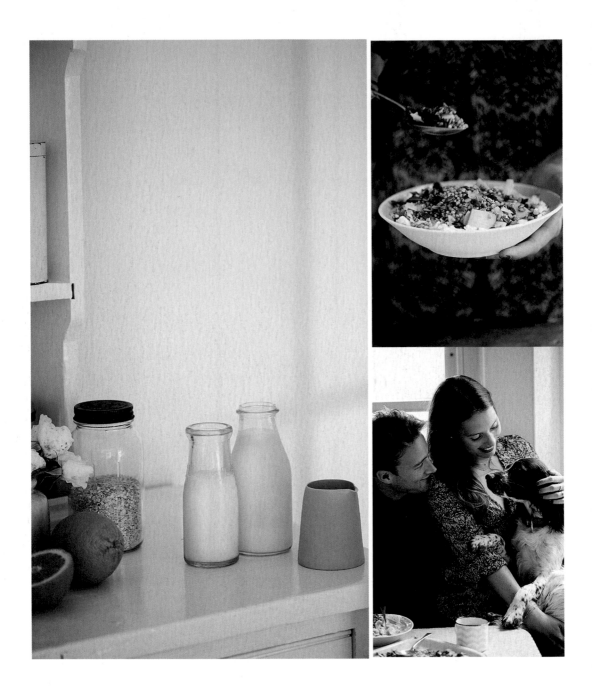

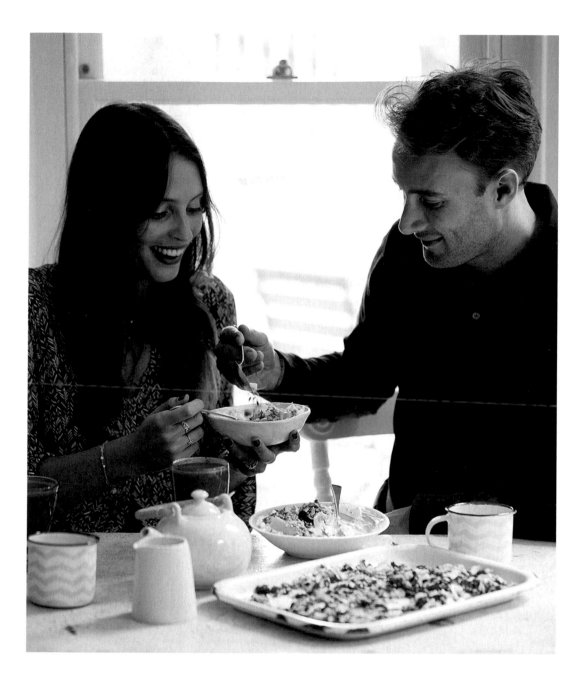

BLUEBERRY PANCAKE STACK

This was one of the first recipes I created for this book, and it is still one of my favorites. I started cooking these to fuel my running when I was training for a half marathon, and they've become a weekend staple ever since. A thick stack of them is my dream breakfast, especially when they're piled high with Caramelized Banana Bites, some extra maple syrup and a big dollop of homemade Crunchy Cacao & Almond Butter (pages 37 and 40). There's really nothing about these that tastes healthy; they feel totally delicious and indulgent.

Makes about 12

2 tablespoons chia seeds

2½ cups rolled oats

2 overripe bananas

3 tablespoons maple syrup

2 tablespoons coconut oil,
   plus more to cook

pinch of salt

1 cup blueberries

Start by putting the chia seeds into a mug with ¾ cup water. Let this sit for 20 minutes until the seeds expand and form a gel.

Place all the other ingredients, except the blueberries and the chia mixture, into a food processor with a scant ½ cup water and blend until you have a smooth batter.

Transfer the mixture to a bowl and stir in the blueberries, then the chia gel.

Oil a nonstick frying pan with a little coconut oil. Place over high heat until it's really hot.

Now simply add 2 heaping tablespoons of batter to the pan for each pancake, use a spoon to shape into an even round and let it cook for about 2 minutes per side, flipping it over once. Repeat for each pancake, until all the batter has been used, keeping them warm in a low oven until you're ready to eat.

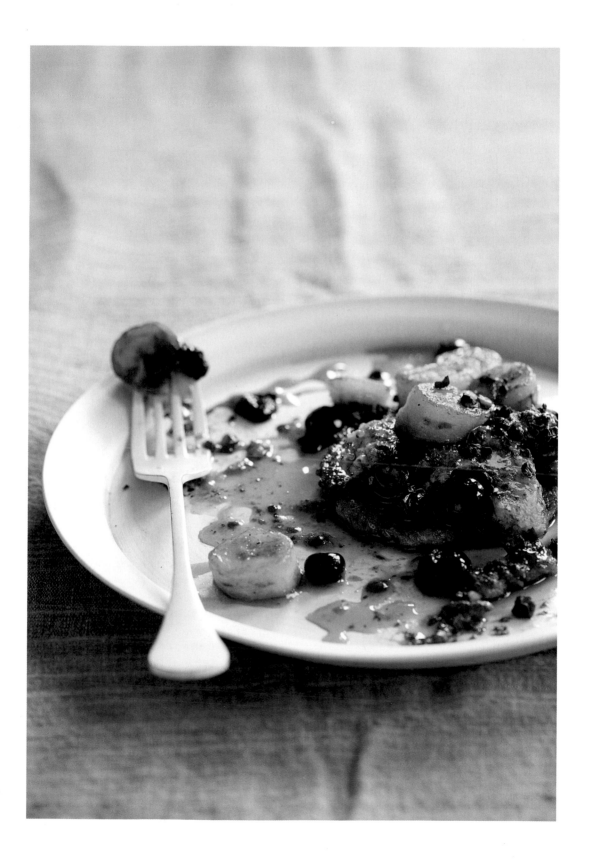

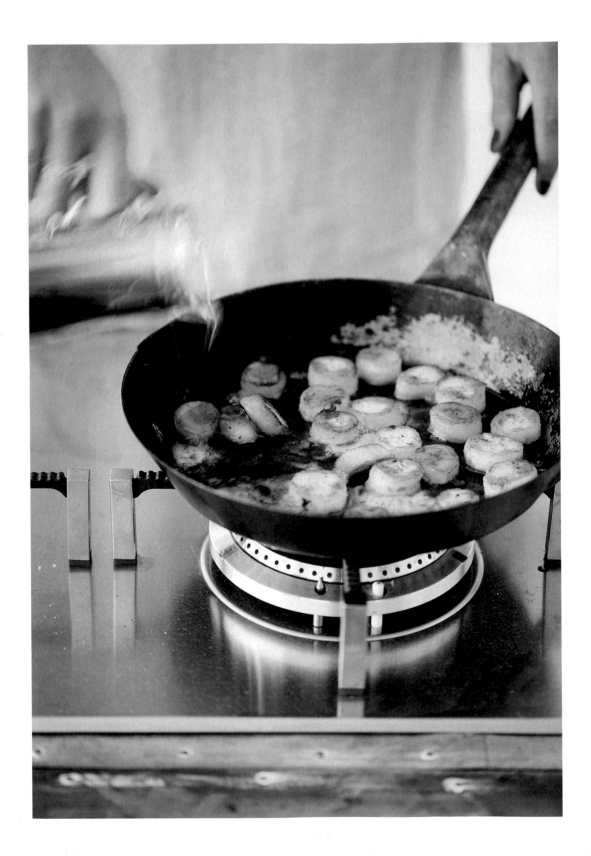

CARAMELIZED BANANA BITES

I made these to enjoy with my Blueberry Pancake Stack (page 34), but loved them so much that I now try to sneak them into my breakfasts all the time. I love how they sizzle in the pan as you fry them, and you can smell the sweet coconut, cinnamon and maple flavors that they're absorbing—it's amazing—plus they're so quick to make. You have to try them with the pancakes, but also experiment by adding these to a simple bowl of oatmeal: they'll instantly transform it into something really special.

Serves 4

4 bananas
1 tablespoon coconut oil
3 tablespoons maple syrup
1 teaspoon ground cinnamon

Slice the bananas into generous ¾-inch-thick slices.

Heat a frying pan with the coconut oil, maple syrup and cinnamon over medium-high heat until it is all really hot and bubbling. Add the banana slices; they should sizzle the moment they hit the pan.

Reduce the heat and cook for 2–3 minutes, stirring occasionally to make sure the slices are all fully coated and cooking evenly. When they're done they should be soft, gooey and coated in caramelized deliciousness!

SUPER SPEEDY
10 minutes

CLEVER COOKING
If you're making these to serve with the pancakes (page 34), then just use the same pan to cook the bananas once you've finished making the pancakes. Cuts down on the cleanup!

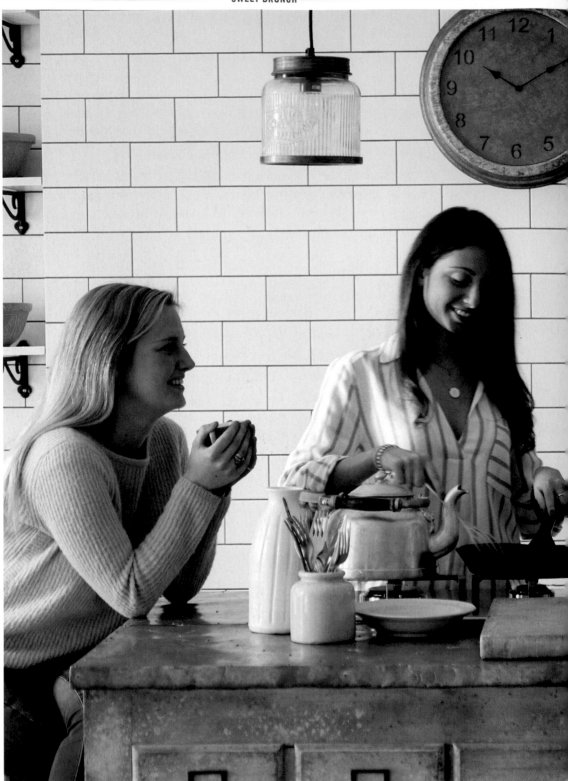

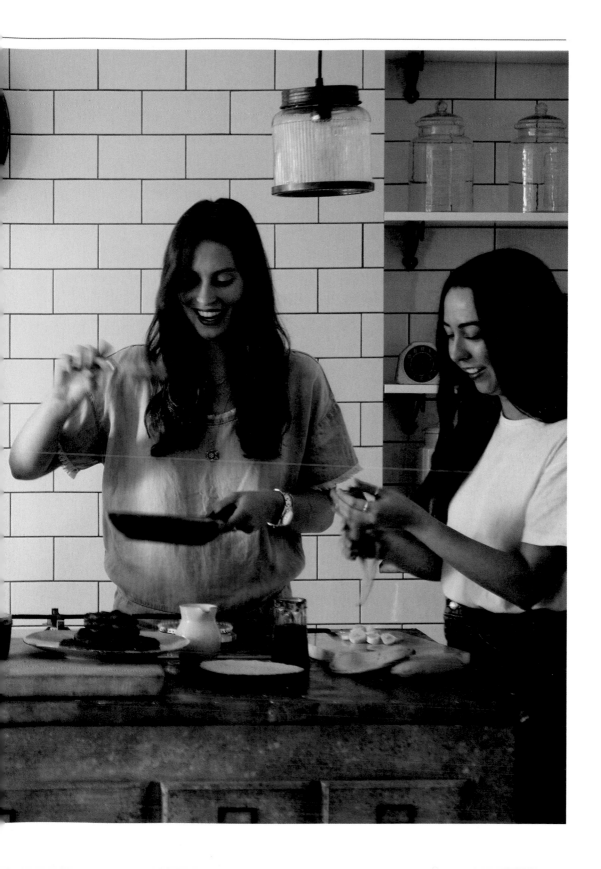

CRUNCHY CACAO & ALMOND BUTTER

Nut butter is a real staple in my life. I always have about ten open jars in my cupboard and at least one spoonful seems to somehow work its way into almost every meal I eat! This is my favorite for breakfast, though; it's got a lovely subtle sweetness from the vanilla, while the cacao nibs give it a great little crunch. Dollop this on pancake stacks, stir it into oatmeal, spread it on toast, blend it into smoothies or just spoon it straight from the jar!

Makes 1 jar

2 cups almonds
generous pinch of salt
4 teaspoons cacao nibs
1 tablespoon raw cacao powder
2 teaspoons date syrup
2 teaspoons vanilla powder

Preheat the oven to 400°F. Spread the almonds over a baking sheet in a single layer and bake for 10 minutes. Keep an eye on them and don't let them burn, as this will ruin the flavors.

Let the almonds cool, then blend with the salt in a high-powered blender for about 10 minutes to form a smooth, creamy paste.

Scrape the almond butter from the blender into a large mixing bowl and stir in all the other ingredients. (Stirring these in, rather than blending, creates a smoother texture.)

Store in an airtight container for up to 5 days.

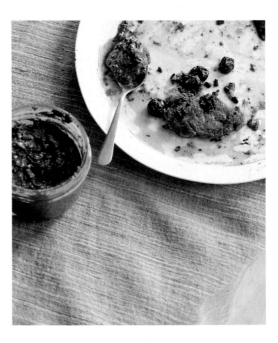

CLEVER COOKING
Make sure the almonds are fresh. All nuts can turn rancid quite quickly in the cupboard, which really affects the taste.

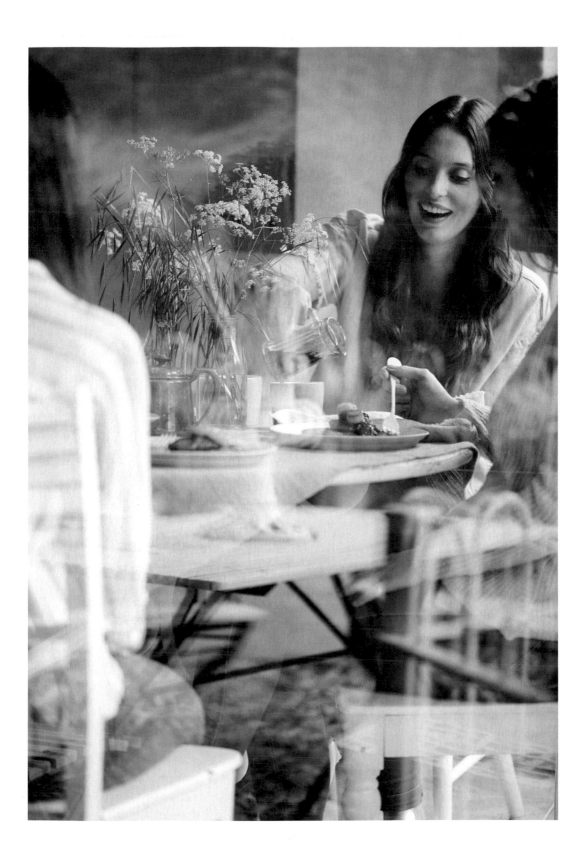

SCRAMBLED TURMERIC & RED PEPPER TOFU

Scrambled tofu might sound really weird, but trust me, it's so worth trying! It makes a lovely breakfast, especially with hot Thyme Fried Mushrooms, Garlicky Baked Tomatoes (pages 45 and 46) and some toasted rye bread spread with a thick layer of smashed avocado.

Serves 4

NUT-FREE

olive oil

1 red bell pepper, finely chopped

6 green onions

¾ ounce chives

1 tablespoon nutritional yeast

1 tablespoon tamari

1 teaspoon ground turmeric

juice of ½ lemon

salt and pepper

14 ounces firm tofu (ideally organic)

SUPER SPEEDY

15 minutes

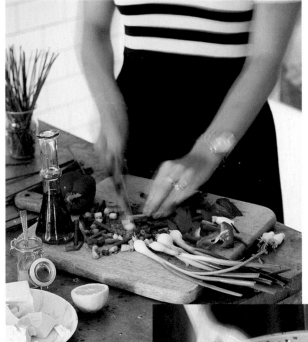

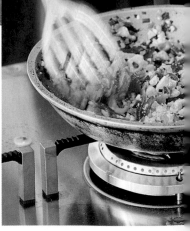

Heat a glug of olive oil in a frying pan and cook the bell pepper for 4–5 minutes.

Meanwhile, finely slice the green onions and chives. Stir the green onions into the peppers and cook for another minute before adding the chives, nutritional yeast, tamari, turmeric, lemon juice and salt and black pepper to taste. Finally, crumble in the tofu.

Cook for another 5 minutes, stirring every now and again, to heat the tofu through.

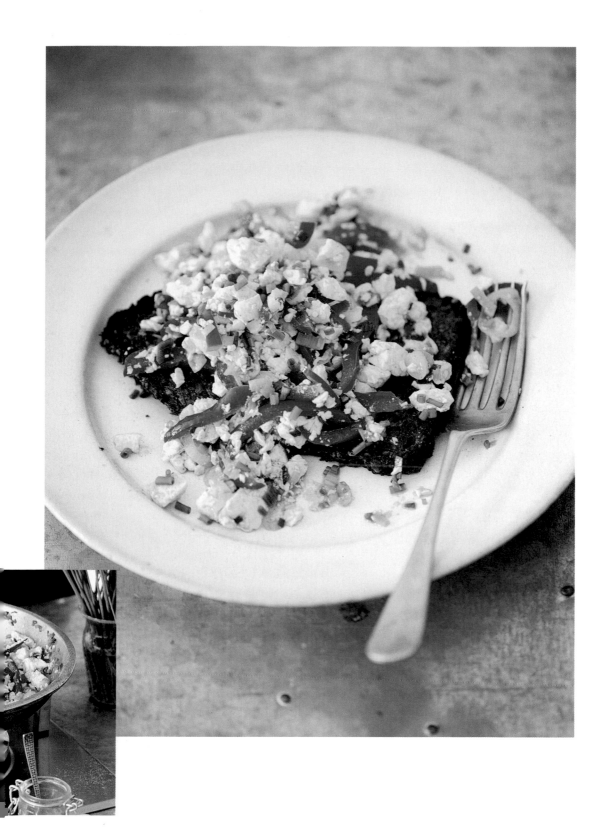

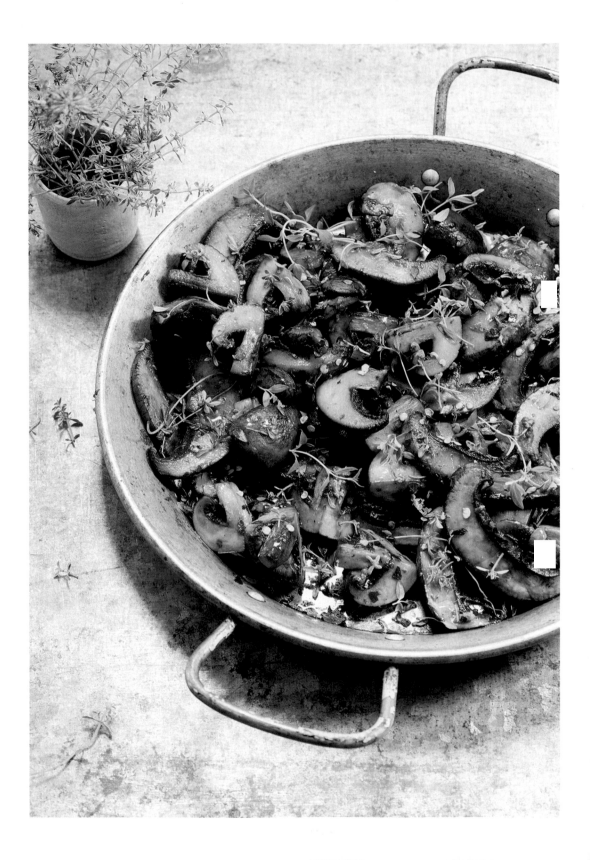

THYME FRIED MUSHROOMS

These are a weekend staple in our house. They're simple to make but bursting with flavor, and make any meal extra satisfying and hearty. I love piling these onto a piece of rye toast with Garlicky Baked Tomatoes (page 46), or using them as a side for a quinoa bowl later in the day.

Serves 4

NUT-FREE

2 garlic cloves, crushed

salt and pepper

olive oil

a few sprigs of fresh thyme

1 teaspoon brown rice miso paste

½ teaspoon chili flakes

6 portobello mushrooms, thickly sliced

12 ounces cremini mushrooms, halved or quartered, depending on size

Place the garlic, salt and pepper in a large frying pan with a glug of olive oil. Let this heat for a few minutes, until it starts bubbling.

Now throw in the thyme and add the miso paste, chili flakes and all the mushrooms. Keep stirring the mushrooms until they release their juices, then let simmer over low heat until most of the juices evaporate.

After about 10 minutes they should be cooked perfectly. Remove from the heat and grind over a good amount of black pepper. Eat straightaway.

SUPER SPEEDY

15 minutes

GARLICKY BAKED TOMATOES

This is a wonderfully simple dish. I find tomatoes often taste best when left mostly untouched, as their natural flavor and juicy texture are really special, especially when baked. Adding the garlic, basil and apple cider vinegar does heighten their natural taste though, which is lovely. An easy addition to any savory breakfast.

Serves 4

NUT-FREE

4 large vine tomatoes

2 tablespoons olive oil

salt and pepper

6 garlic cloves, peeled

¾ pound cherry tomatoes, preferably on the vine

2 tablespoons apple cider vinegar

small handful of basil leaves

Preheat the oven to 400°F.

While the oven heats up, cut the vine tomatoes in half. Place them flat sides down on a rimmed baking sheet and drizzle with the olive oil. Grind on lots of salt and pepper and throw in the whole garlic cloves.

Bake for 30 minutes.

Take the tomatoes out of the oven and add the cherry tomatoes and vinegar. Reduce the oven temperature to 350°F and bake all the tomatoes together for another 40–45 minutes.

Roughly chop or tear the basil and sprinkle over the tomatoes and garlic before serving.

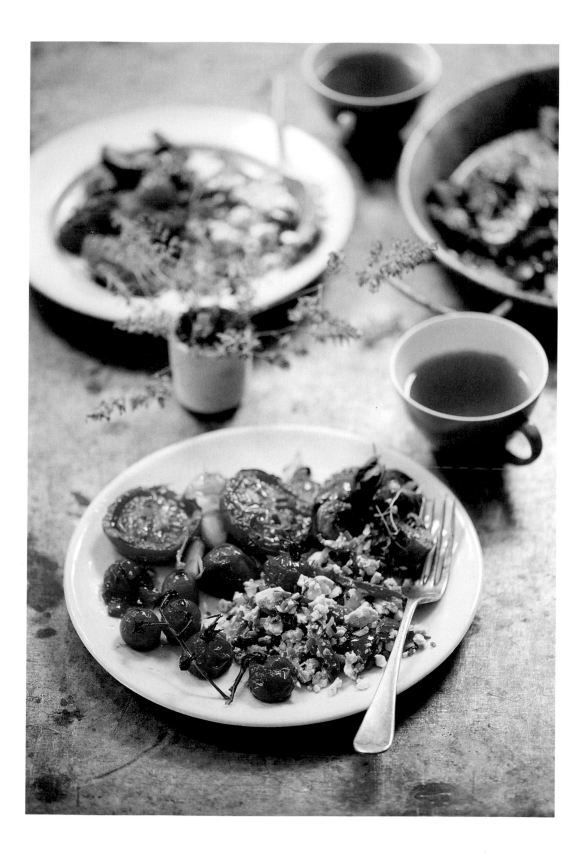

SWEET POTATO RÖSTI

A great base for a big breakfast. I love spreading a thick layer of my Herby Guacamole on top of these, then piling them high with hot Maple & Rosemary Butter Beans (pages 52 and 51). It makes for a really beautiful, hearty and delicious brunch.

Serves 2

NUT-FREE

4 tablespoons olive oil

1 sweet potato, peeled and grated

1 fresh red chile, seeded and finely chopped (if you like it less spicy, only use ½ chile)

1 tablespoon sesame seeds

¼ cup buckwheat flour

salt and pepper

In a large, nonstick lidded frying pan, heat 2 tablespoons of the oil over high heat.

Meanwhile, place the remaining ingredients in a bowl and mix them thoroughly.

Spoon the sweet potato mixture into the hot oil, in 4 even mounds, making sure they're not touching each other. Cook over high heat for about 2 minutes, gently pressing the mixture down every now and again so that they compress into nicely shaped patties.

Cover the pan and reduce the heat to as low as it will go. Let the steam cook the patties through for about 7 minutes. When you take the lid off, the underside of the röstis should be lovely and crispy and the patties will have reduced in size.

Add the remaining 2 tablespoons of oil and gently turn the röstis over with a spatula. Whack the heat up to high again and cook for 3 minutes, or until the second side is browned nicely. Serve hot.

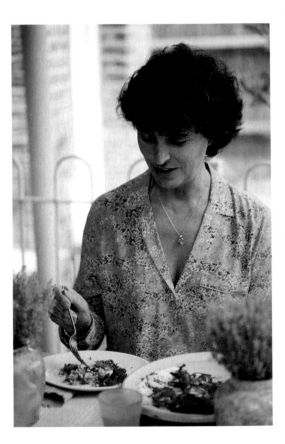

PAN TO PLATE

20 minutes

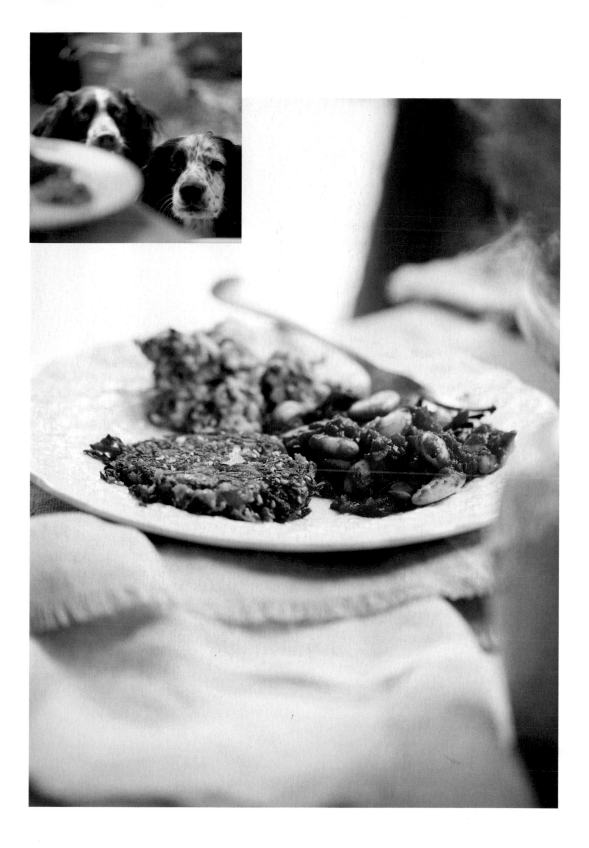

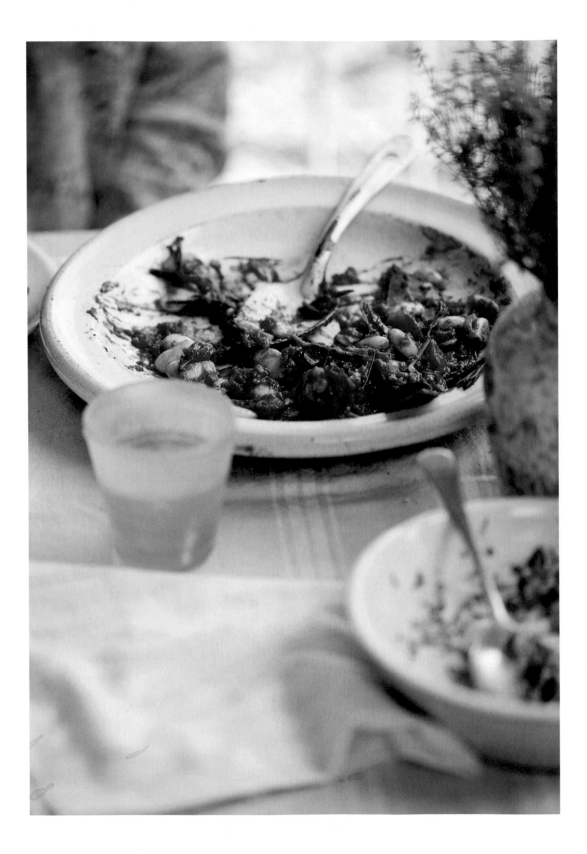

MAPLE & ROSEMARY BUTTER BEANS

In our house, we seem to find ways to include these in breakfast, lunch and dinner!
They're so versatile and go with just about everything, although they are especially good
in this brunch combination. I just love how simple and yet how flavorful they are.

Serves 2

NUT-FREE

olive oil

3 garlic cloves, finely chopped

3 sprigs of fresh rosemary

1 bay leaf

½ teaspoon cayenne pepper

1 teaspoon smoked paprika

½ cup canned diced tomatoes (about ⅓ can)

1 tablespoon maple syrup

1 tablespoon tomato paste

one 15-ounce can butter beans (or lima beans),
    drained and rinsed

salt and pepper

Preheat the oven to 350°F.

Use a Dutch oven for this dish. Heat up a glug of olive oil and fry the garlic over medium heat until it turns translucent but doesn't color. Once this happens, add the herbs and spices, tomatoes, maple syrup and tomato paste, the beans, salt and pepper. Bring to a boil.

Once it starts to boil, clamp the lid on, transfer the pan to the oven and bake for 30 minutes.

Remove the bay leaf and rosemary stems before serving (the rosemary leaves will have dropped off into the beans) and enjoy.

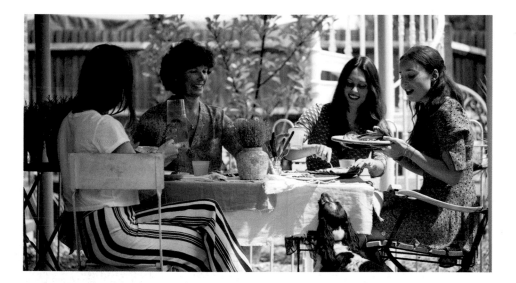

HERBY GUACAMOLE

*Probably my favorite part of this brunch, with the rösti and butter beans (pages 48
and 51). I find that the creamy texture really brings the other two dishes together.
The avocado is mixed with a beautiful blend of roughly chopped aromatic basil,
cilantro, mint and parsley, to create something that's just bursting with flavor;
I'm sure all you avocado fans will absolutely love it! It's a great addition
to any meal. I adore piling it onto a slice of rye toast for breakfast,
using it as a dip for a quick snack or adding it to a big quinoa bowl.*

Serves 2

NUT-FREE

2 avocados
1 tablespoon olive oil
juice of 1 lime
¼ cup fresh basil leaves, roughly
   chopped
¼ cup cilantro leaves, roughly chopped
2 tablespoons fresh mint leaves,
   roughly chopped
2 tablespoons fresh parsley leaves,
   roughly chopped
lots of salt and pepper

Pit and peel the avocados, then mash
them in a bowl with a fork.

Stir in all the rest of the ingredients. This is
best served fresh. It won't keep for more
than a day or so and the herbs will start to
turn brown.

SUPER SPEEDY
10 minutes

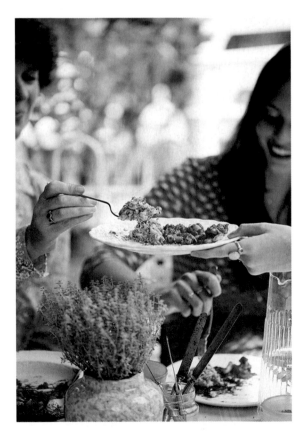

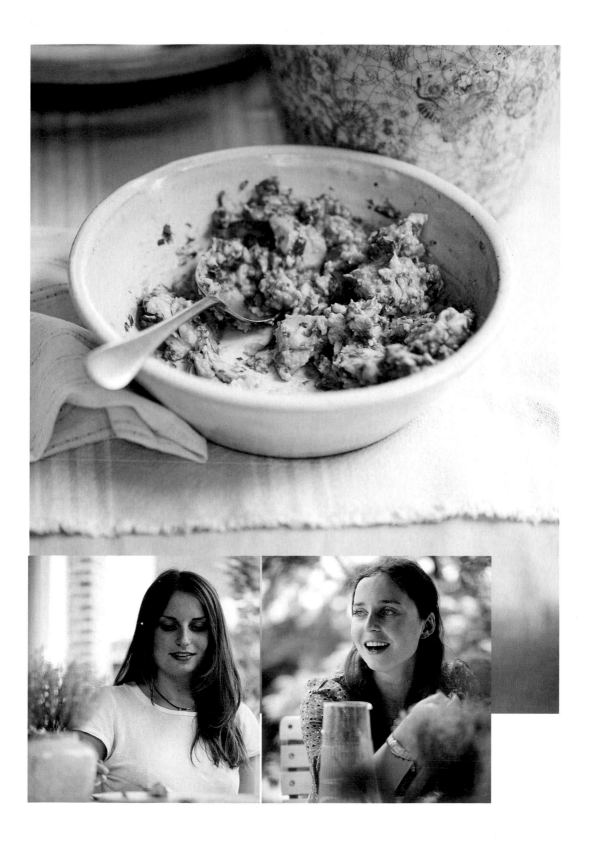

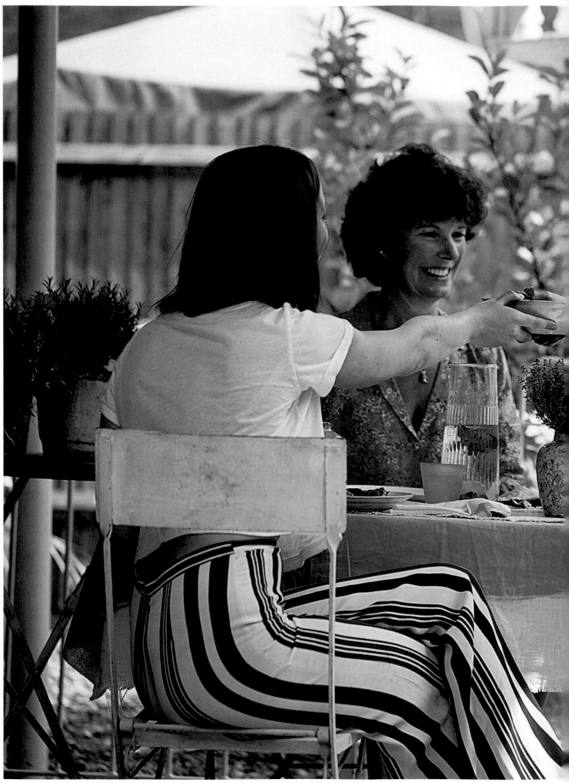

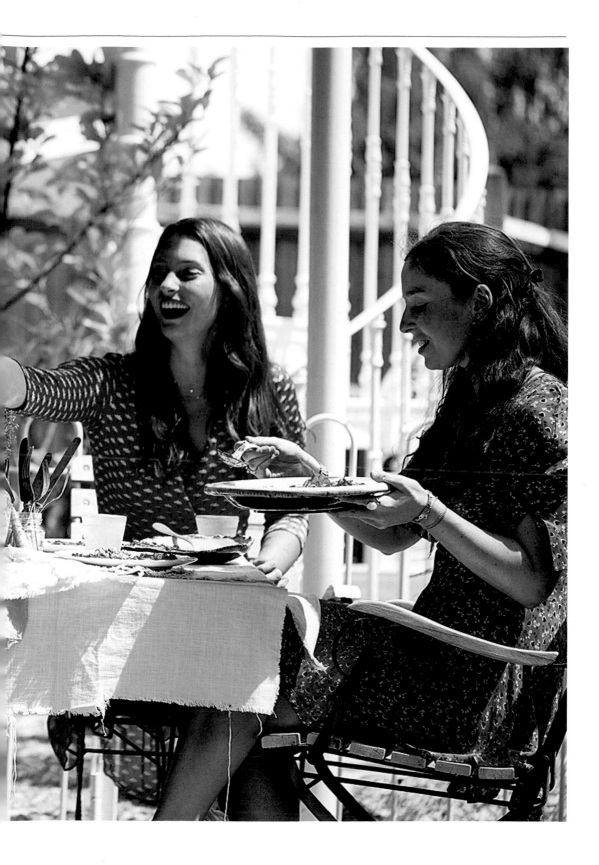

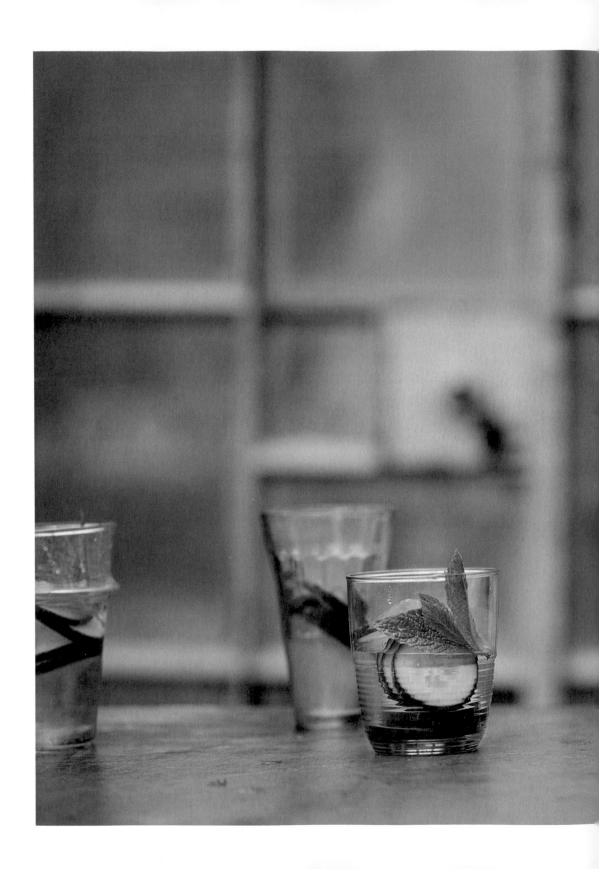

LIGHT & EASY

QUICK MEALS TO NOURISH YOUR BODY & FEED YOUR FRIENDS

LIGHT & EASY

This is probably the chapter of the book that I use the most at home. It's packed with simple recipes that you can make and share every day, to keep you and the people around you feeling happy and healthy. It's hard to pick favorites from these recipes, as I genuinely love and use them all, but I would recommend a plate of hot Spiced Potato Cakes with Garlicky Tomato Sauce on a bed of Haricots Verts with Tomato if you want something nourishing and warming, or the Mango & Mushroom Ceviche if you want something lighter and more refreshing. Or, if you're looking for an upgrade to your lunch box, or to put together a simple picnic to share with a friend, try the Kale, Sun-Dried Tomato, Olive & Sweet Potato Salad with Baked Sweet Potato & Sesame Falafels and maybe a side of hummus.

MENUS

AFTER-WORK CATCH-UP
Spiced Potato Cakes with Garlicky Tomato Sauce
Haricots Verts with Tomato

FRESH BITES
Mango & Mushroom Ceviche
Cauli Rice, Sesame & Beet Nigiri Sushi

AL DESKO
Baked Sweet Potato & Sesame Falafels
Kale, Sun-Dried Tomato, Olive & Sweet Potato Salad

PERFECT PICNIC
Charred Coconut Corn
Pepper, Mango, Cucumber & Peanut Salad

PANTRY SAVIOR
Lemony Potato & Butter Bean Salad
Baked Sesame & Tomato Avocados

COMFORT & SPICE
Sweet Potato Noodles with a Creamy Peanut Satay Sauce
Sautéed Tamari Greens

ASIAN-STYLE SUPPER
Chile & Ginger Pho
Sesame & Maple Summer Rolls with Sweet Almond Dipping Sauce

SUMMER SALADS
Pistachio & Apricot Quinoa
Sesame Slaw

MIDWEEK PICK-ME-UP
Sautéed Tempeh with Roasted Garlic & Almond Pesto
Sesame, Cilantro & Roasted Fennel Rice Bowl

SPICED POTATO CAKES WITH GARLICKY TOMATO SAUCE

These make an excellent weekday dinner. They're easy to make and so comforting after a long day at work, especially when covered in piping hot garlicky tomato sauce and served on a bed of green beans that echo their flavors (page 65). The potato cakes have so much flavor themselves, with their warming mix of spices and lemon, which adds a lovely freshness. Freeze any leftover cakes.

Makes 8 / Serves 4

NUT-FREE

FOR THE POTATO CAKES

1⅔ pounds potatoes

salt and pepper

3 tablespoons olive oil, plus more to drizzle

1 fresh red chile, seeded and finely
    chopped, plus more to serve

2 garlic cloves, crushed

1 teaspoon ground cumin

1 teaspoon paprika

1 teaspoon ground turmeric

1 teaspoon chili powder

½ cup cilantro, roughly chopped,
    plus more to serve

juice of 1 lemon

FOR THE SAUCE

1 pound 10 ounces cherry tomatoes,
    quartered

3 tablespoons olive oil

4 garlic cloves, crushed

1 teaspoon chili flakes (optional)

salt and pepper

Peel the potatoes, quarter them, then place them in a saucepan of water with a pinch of salt. Bring to a boil and simmer for 20–25 minutes, until cooked. Drain and let cool.

Meanwhile, heat the 3 tablespoons oil in a frying pan, add the chile and garlic and cook for a minute or so. Add the dry spices, sizzle for 30 seconds, then remove from the heat. Preheat the oven to 400°F.

Once the potatoes have cooled, add the chile/spice oil, the cilantro and lemon juice. Mix until smooth, then shape into 8 patties. Place on a baking sheet. Drizzle with olive oil. Bake for 25–30 minutes, turning halfway, until they are golden brown.

Meanwhile, make the sauce. Simply throw all the ingredients into a saucepan and simmer for about 20 minutes, or until the tomatoes have cooked down and the sauce is rich and thick.

Serve the potato cakes with the sauce, sprinkling with cilantro and chopped chile, with the Haricots Verts with Tomato (page 65).

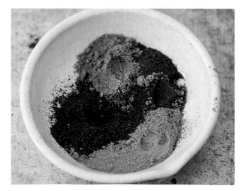

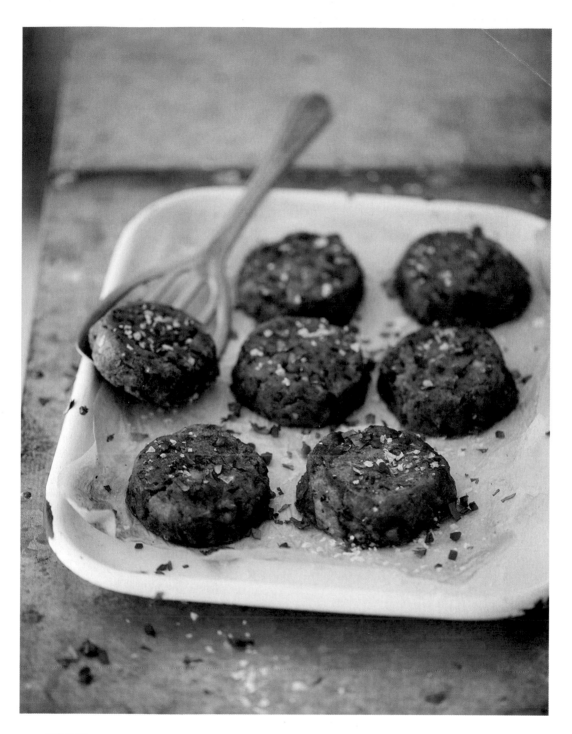

MIX IT UP

If you want to skip the tomato sauce, these potato cakes also taste incredible with Coconut Tzatziki (page 209).

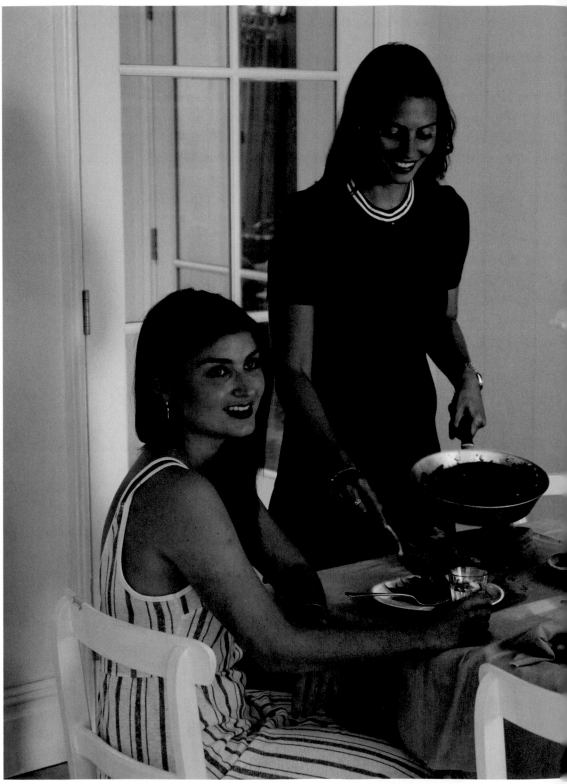

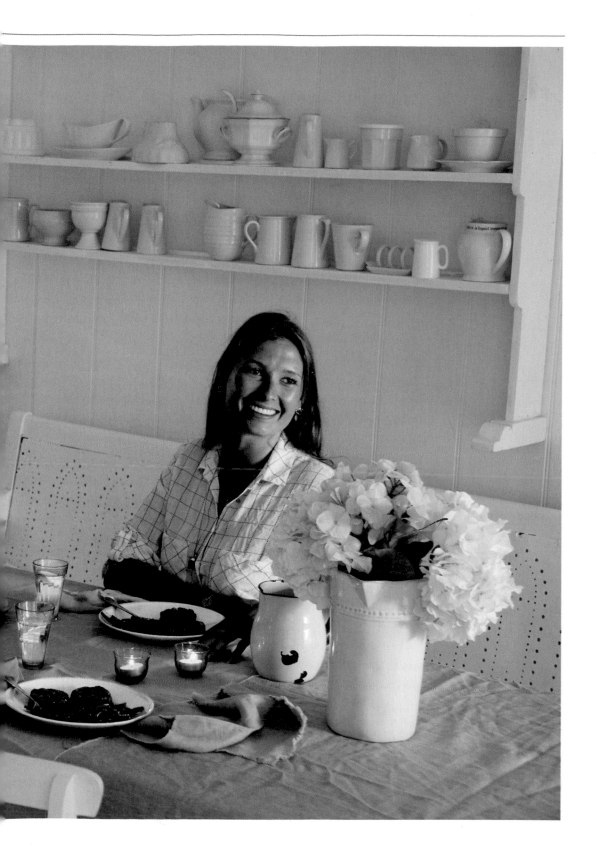

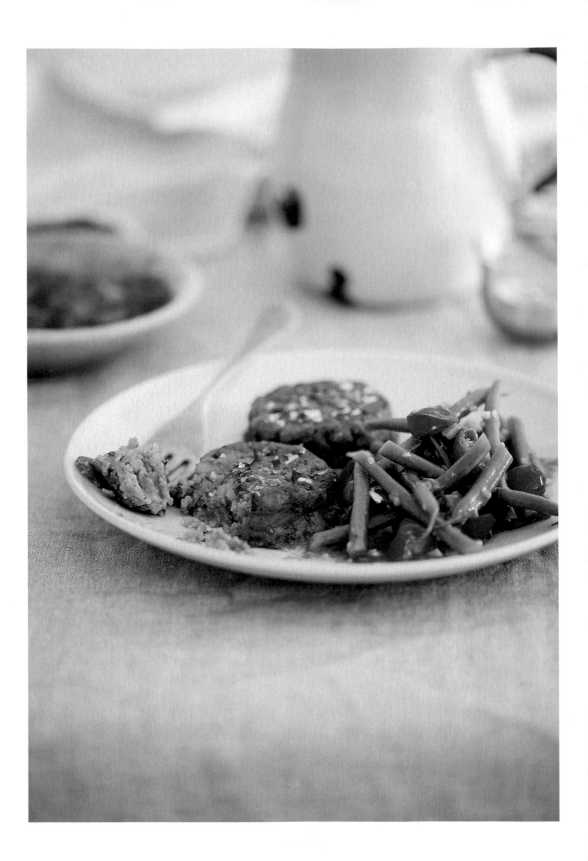

HARICOTS VERTS WITH TOMATO

I love using these as a bed for my Spiced Potato Cakes with Garlicky Tomato Sauce (page 60), as the contrast of textures is so perfect. The lightly cooked beans have a lovely snap and crunch, while the potato cakes are soft and just melt in your mouth. The garlic and tomato in the beans really complement the sauce of the potatoes, too, creating a perfect meal. These beans work as a great side with a host of other meals.

Serves 4 as a side dish

NUT-FREE

2 tablespoons olive oil

4 ounces cherry tomatoes, quartered

3 garlic cloves, crushed

1 tablespoon apple cider vinegar

salt and pepper

½ pound haricots verts, tops trimmed, halved

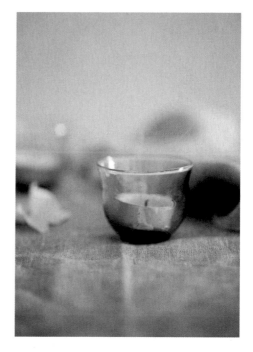

Heat the olive oil in a large sauté pan over medium heat. Add the tomatoes and let them cook down until they start to disintegrate and caramelize. Meanwhile fill a kettle with water and bring it to a boil.

When the tomatoes are a rich red color, after about 5 minutes, add the garlic, vinegar and salt and pepper to taste and cook for about 1 minute.

Meanwhile, pop the green beans into a sieve and pour the boiling water from the kettle over them so they start to soften, then put them into the pan with the tomato and garlic mixture.

Stir over the heat for a couple of minutes to heat through, season to taste, then serve.

SUPER SPEEDY

15 minutes

MIX IT UP

Try stirring these into a bowl of penne pasta; it's absolutely delicious and a wonderfully quick meal.

MANGO & MUSHROOM CEVICHE

I first had a mushroom ceviche at one of my favorite restaurants about a year ago and have been in love with the dish ever since. It's wonderfully light, full of flavor and incredibly refreshing. The mushrooms are marinated in an amazing mix of lime juice, ginger, chile and olive oil, then tossed with juicy bites of mango and crunchy red bell pepper, which together taste incredible. The flavors only get stronger the longer you marinate this, so make extra to enjoy as leftovers a few days later.

Serves 4

NUT-FREE

14 ounces button mushrooms, very
   thinly sliced
⅔ cup lime juice (about 10 limes)
scant ¼ cup olive oil
1 garlic clove, crushed
1 inch fresh ginger, finely grated
1 jalapeño, or other fresh chile,
   finely chopped
salt
⅓ red onion, finely chopped
1 red bell pepper, finely chopped
¾ mango, peeled, pitted and
   finely chopped
small handful of cilantro,
   roughly chopped

Place the mushrooms in a large bowl and pour over the lime juice, olive oil, garlic, ginger, jalapeño and salt to taste. Toss together gently, cover and marinate for 1 hour at room temperature for the flavors to develop.

When you're ready to serve, stir in the onion, bell pepper, mango and most of the cilantro, then arrange it on a serving platter. Sprinkle on the remaining cilantro when you serve, to make it look even more beautiful.

Any leftovers will keep in an airtight container in the fridge for up to 4 days.

SUPER SPEEDY
10 minutes

MIX IT UP
Try topping this with the kernels cut from Charred Coconut Corn (page 76). It tastes amazing.

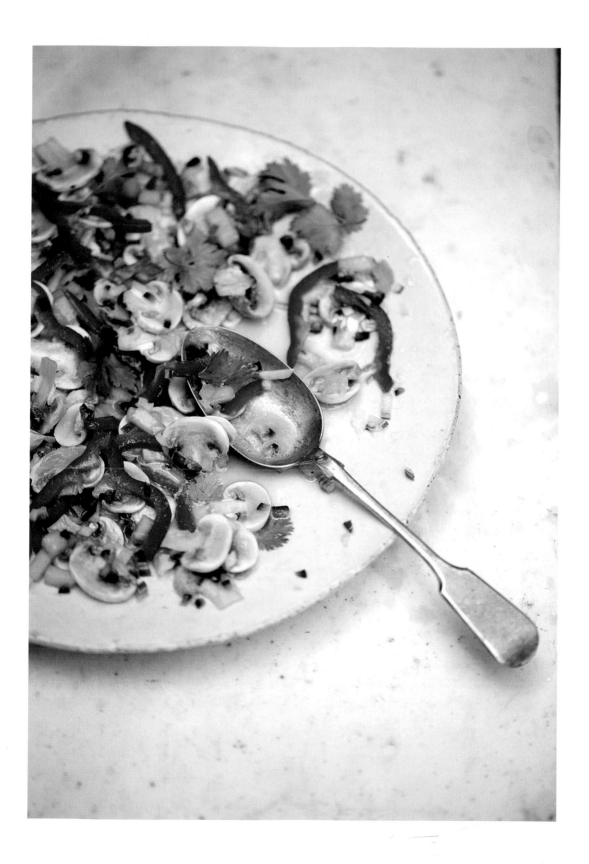

CAULI RICE, SESAME & BEET NIGIRI SUSHI

This veggie nigiri is a little unusual and it's a really lovely nibble. Using cauliflower rice makes a nice, light change from sushi rice, while the brightly colored avocado and beet make it look fantastic. I love dipping these nigiri into the tamari, sesame and lime sauce, to deepen the flavors. You'll need a jelly bag to prepare the rice; find them online.

Makes 10 pieces

FOR THE "RICE"

1 large head cauliflower

1 tablespoon apple cider vinegar

1 tablespoon toasted sesame oil

1 tablespoon tamari

½ cup coconut milk

salt

FOR THE AVOCADO CREAM

1 avocado

1 tablespoon apple cider vinegar

1 tablespoon olive oil

FOR THE BEET

1 beet, cooked and peeled

FOR THE DIPPING SAUCE

juice of ½ lime

2 tablespoons tamari

1 tablespoon sesame oil

1 tablespoon sesame seeds,
    plus more to serve

Cut the cauliflower florets from the stem and chop them into 1–2-inch pieces. This will make "ricing" them easier. Place in a food processor and pulse until it looks like rice; this takes about 30 seconds.

Place in a jelly bag and knead out excess water. This takes a few minutes as cauliflower contains a lot of water. It's a really important step though, so please don't skip it, or the rice won't hold together when you mold it.

Once most of the water has been removed, add the cauliflower to a saucepan with the remaining rice ingredients and simmer over medium heat for about 10 minutes, or until the coconut milk has been absorbed and there is no liquid left in the pan. The rice should start to feel a bit sticky at this point. Put it into a sieve and press out any remaining liquid, then tip it out into a bowl and firmly press it down. Set aside.

Now make the avocado cream. Scoop the avocado flesh into a food processor with all the remaining avocado cream ingredients, adding 1 tablespoon water and a little salt. Blend until the mixture is smooth and creamy. Set aside.

Very finely slice the beet.

To make the dipping sauce, simply mix all the ingredients together thoroughly.

Now assemble the nigiri. Mold the cauliflower rice into little oblong nigiri shapes. Spoon a neat blob of the avocado cream on top and lay a thin slice of beet over the cream. Sprinkle with sesame seeds, then arrange on a serving platter with shallow bowls of the dipping sauce.

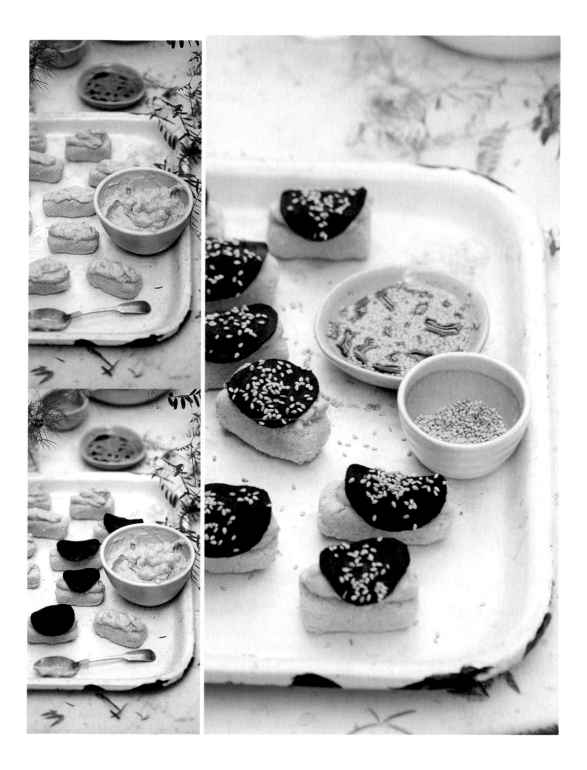

BAKED SWEET POTATO & SESAME FALAFELS

These are such a great addition to an on-the-go lunch box. They're quick and simple to make and freeze well, too, so you can build a stash in the freezer to keep you fueled throughout the week. I love the sesame seeds on the outside; it gives such a lovely crunch and makes them look beautiful. They also travel really easily, making them a great al desko lunch, so I'm sure lots of your colleagues will be very jealous! They taste amazing with Kale, Sun-Dried Tomato, Olive & Sweet Potato Salad (page 75); the contrasting textures are perfect together.

Makes 14

NUT-FREE

FOR THE SWEET POTATO PURÉE

2 sweet potatoes, peeled and
  roughly chopped

FOR THE FALAFELS

4 garlic cloves, roughly chopped

handful of cilantro, chopped

¼ cup olive oil

juice of 1 lemon

2 teaspoons ground cumin

2 teaspoons smoked paprika

1 teaspoon ground turmeric

2 teaspoons apple cider vinegar

½ teaspoon cayenne pepper

2 tablespoons tahini

3 tablespoons chickpea flour

salt and pepper

two 15-ounce cans chickpeas,
  drained and rinsed

⅔ cup sesame seeds

Steam the sweet potatoes for 30 minutes, or until completely soft. Blend for a few seconds to make a smooth purée.

Preheat the oven to 425°F. Line 1 large or 2 medium baking sheets with parchment paper.

Put all the ingredients for the falafels, except the chickpeas and sesame seeds, into a food processor, add ¾ cup plus 2 tablespoons of the sweet potato purée and blend until almost smooth, then season really well, add the chickpeas and pulse a few times to form a chunky mix.

Tip the sesame seeds onto a plate.

With wet hands, roll 1 tablespoon of the mixture into a ball, roll it in the sesame seeds and place it on the baking sheet(s). Keep going until all the mixture is used up.

Place the sheet(s) into the oven and bake for 35–40 minutes, until golden brown. Let cool for 5 minutes on a wire rack before eating.

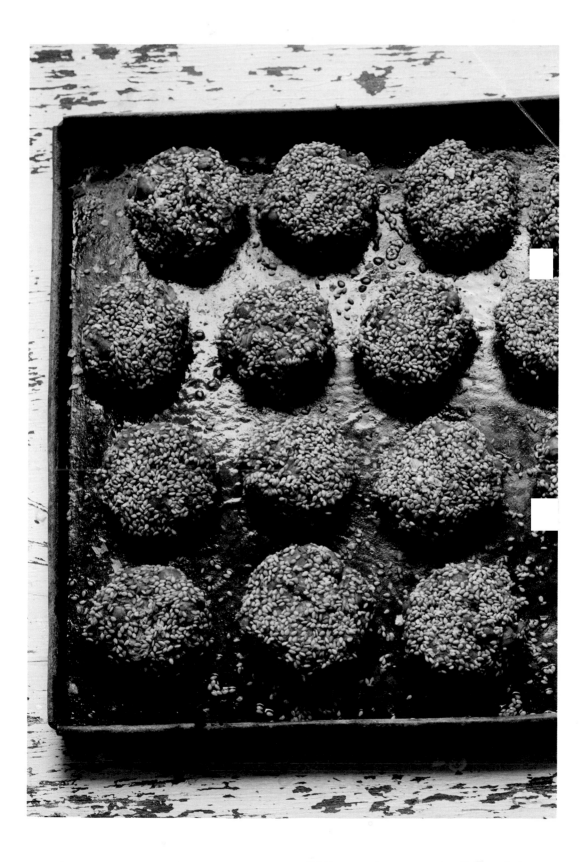

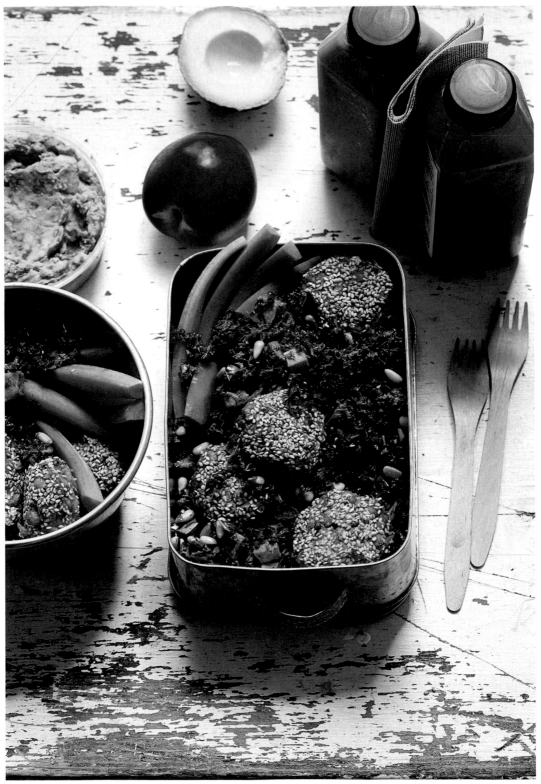

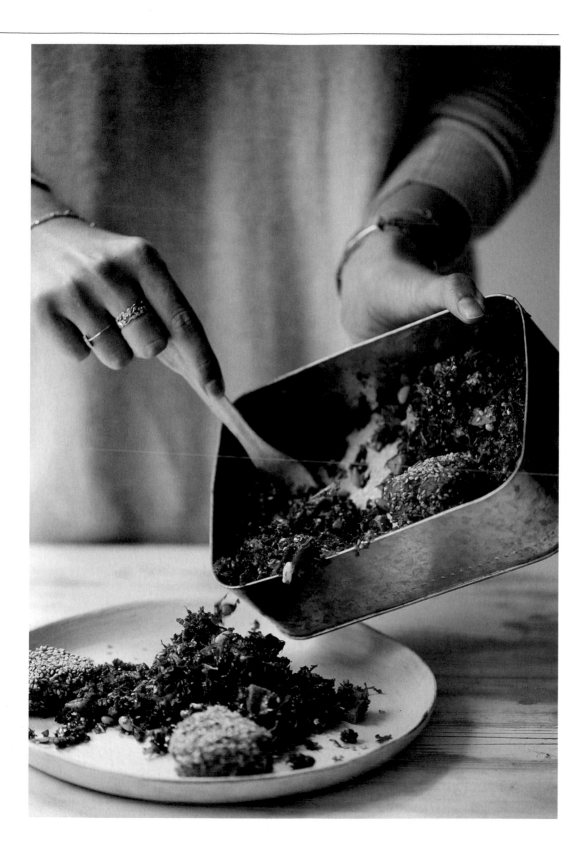

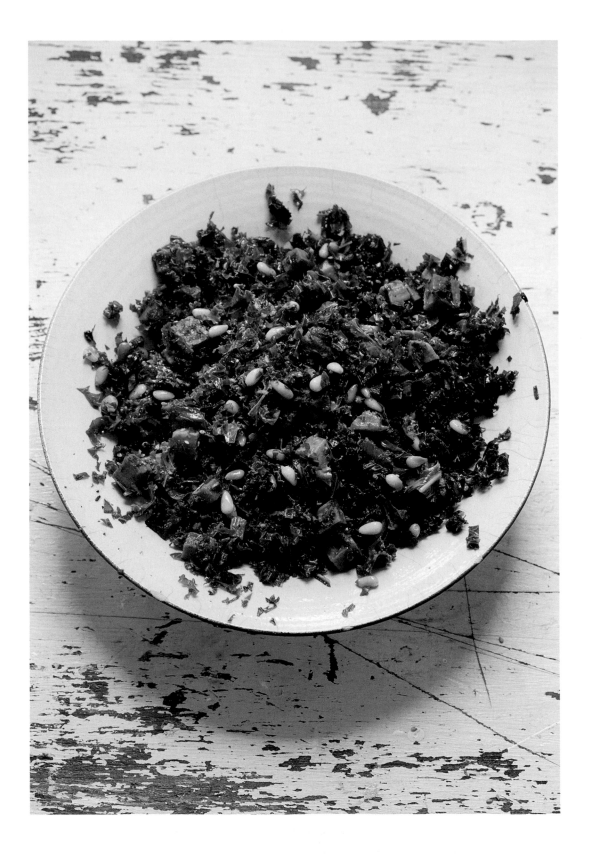

KALE, SUN-DRIED TOMATO, OLIVE & SWEET POTATO SALAD

A lovely chopped salad, filled with little bites of sweet potato, sun-dried tomatoes, black olives and toasted pine nuts, all tossed together with a simple olive oil, lemon and vinegar dressing. Its simplicity means it goes with just about everything, a perfect side salad for every meal! I particularly love it coupled with Baked Sweet Potato & Sesame Falafels (page 70), which makes a fantastic desk lunch, especially with a generous dollop of hummus or guacamole.

Serves 4

NUT-FREE

1 large sweet potato, peeled or
   well scrubbed
5 tablespoons olive oil
salt and pepper
7 ounces kale, coarse ribs removed
2 tablespoons apple cider vinegar
juice of ½ lemon
1 cup oil-packed sun-dried tomatoes
   (3½ ounces drained weight), finely
   chopped
¾ cup pitted black olives, finely chopped
scant ¾ cup pine nuts

Preheat the oven to 425°F.

Cut the sweet potato into ⅓-inch cubes, place on a rimmed baking sheet, drizzle with 2 tablespoons of the olive oil and add lots of salt and pepper. Roast for 45 minutes, or until cooked through and slightly crispy.

Meanwhile, add the kale to a food processor and pulse a few times to break it down into little pieces. Tip it into a large salad bowl with the remaining 3 tablespoons olive oil, the vinegar, lemon juice, sun-dried tomatoes, olives and salt and pepper to taste. Toss well to evenly coat.

When the sweet potato chunks are cooked, remove from the oven and stir them into the salad.

Finally, heat a frying pan over medium heat and dry-fry the pine nuts for a few minutes, or until golden brown. (Watch carefully when cooking these, as they burn easily.) Remove from the heat and sprinkle onto the salad.

This tastes delicious warm or cold.

CHARRED COCONUT CORN

My family has an obsession with coconut corn. We've been eating it nonstop every summer for the last few years. There's something so delicious about the lightly charred corn kernels being coated in sweet coconut oil and salt; it's so addictive! They're amazing made indoors on a grill pan, but if you can cook them on the grill, they're even better.

Serves 4

coconut oil
4 ears of corn, husked
salt

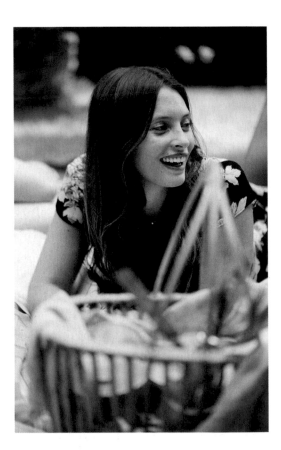

Put a grill pan on the heat with a couple of tablespoons of coconut oil and get it nice and hot. Open the kitchen windows and doors and put on the exhaust fan or—even better—cook it outdoors.

Add the corn. You want to blacken some of the kernels, so leave it well alone for about a minute before you roll it onto another side, making sure you use some tongs, not fingers! Keep doing this until the corn is a nice mixture of black and yellow all round, then remove it and let it cool a little.

Sprinkle with salt and eat.

MIX IT UP
Try cutting the corn kernels off the cob and sprinkling them over Mango & Mushroom Ceviche (page 66); the two recipes taste amazing together!

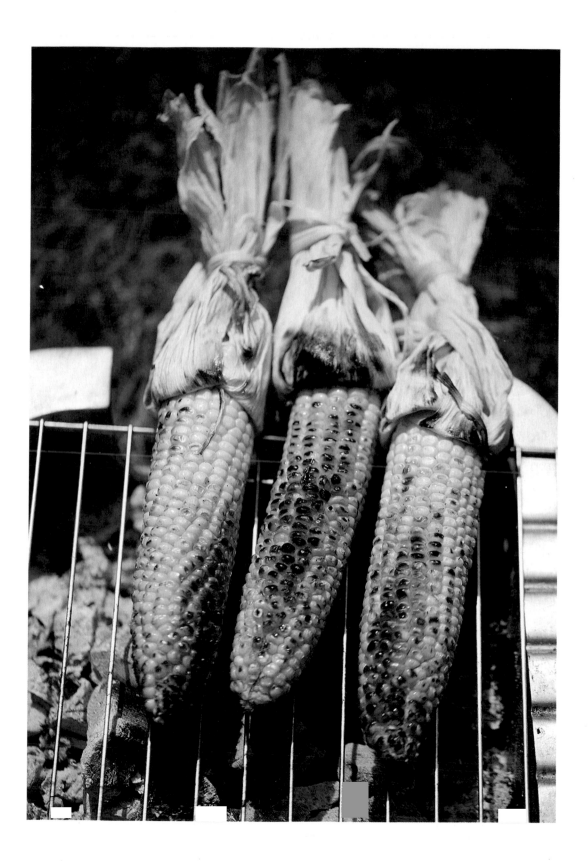

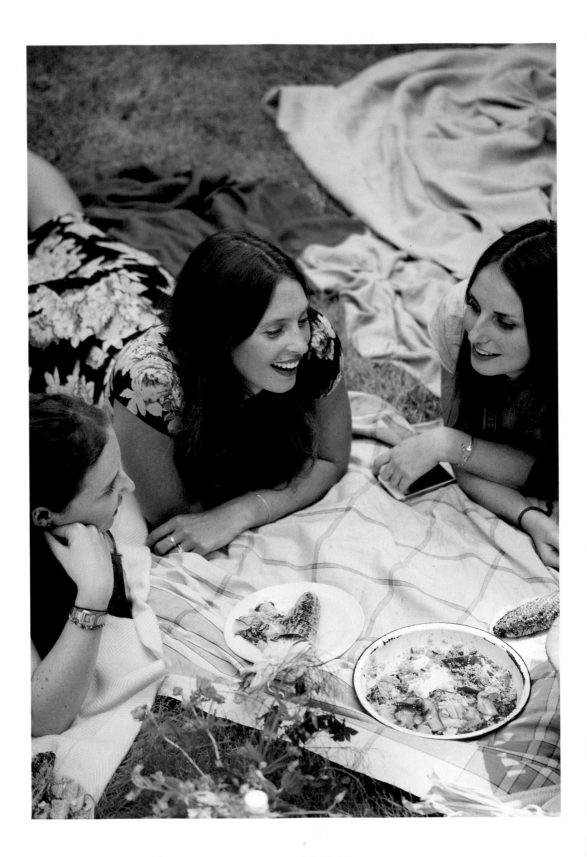

PEPPER, MANGO, CUCUMBER & PEANUT SALAD

A lovely summer lunch. The mango gives each bite a lovely sweetness, while the peanuts and sesame add great texture and flavor. It tastes amazing with kernels of Charred Coconut Corn (page 76) sprinkled across it, too!

Serves 4

FOR THE SALAD

¾ cup unsalted raw peanuts

2 tablespoons sesame seeds

1 red bell pepper, finely sliced

4 garlic cloves, bashed, skins left on

olive oil

scant ¾ cup quinoa

1 small cucumber, shaved into ribbons
   with a peeler

½ fresh red chile, seeded and finely chopped

1 mango, finely chopped

FOR THE DRESSING

2 tablespoons apple cider vinegar

2 tablespoons tamari

2 tablespoons sesame oil

1 tablespoon peanut butter

Preheat the oven to 400°F. Place the peanuts on a rimmed baking sheet and roast for 4 minutes. Give the peanuts a shake, add the sesame seeds and pop them back in the oven for another 4 minutes, or until nicely browned. Set aside to cool.

Tumble the sliced bell pepper onto another baking sheet with the garlic cloves. Drizzle with olive oil and roast for 20 minutes, until soft, giving them a shake halfway through.

Meanwhile, cook the quinoa. Put it into a saucepan with 1 cup water, bring to a boil and simmer for 12–15 minutes, until all the water is absorbed. Set aside to cool. Mix the quinoa and roasted red pepper in a large salad bowl. Pick out the roasted garlic, peel and finely slice it, then stir it in, too.

When you're ready to eat, simply add the peanuts and sesame seeds, cucumber, chile and mango.

Mix all the ingredients for the dressing and toss gently with the salad and devour.

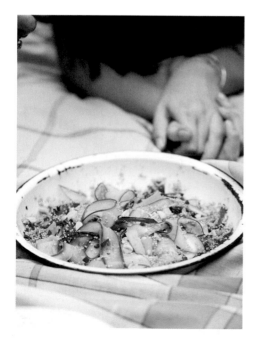

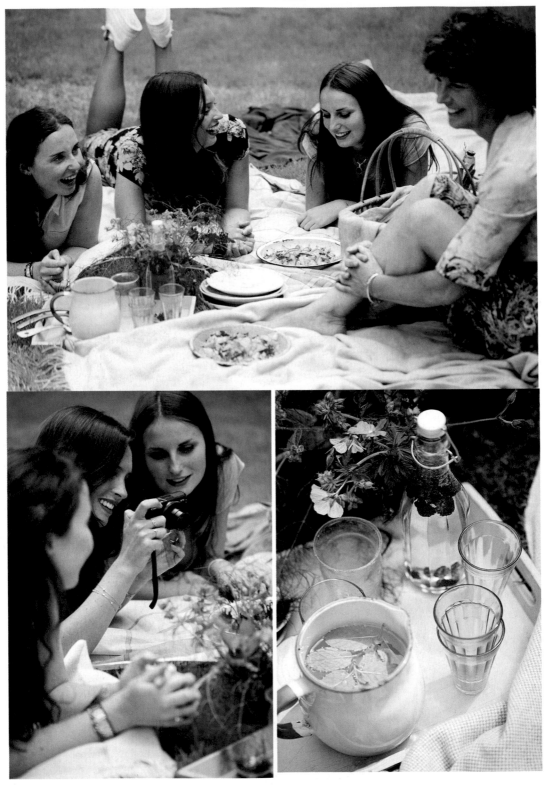

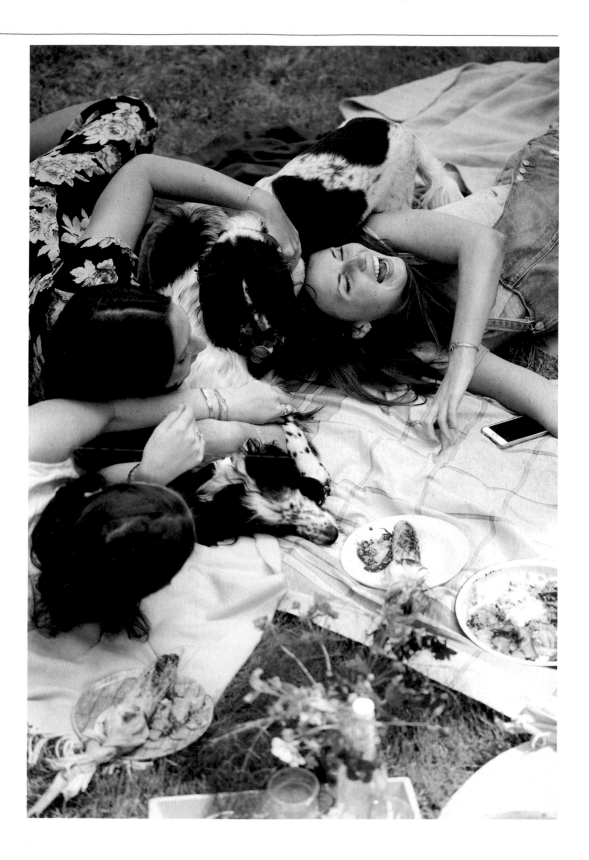

LEMONY POTATO & BUTTER BEAN SALAD

This is the perfect simple salad for a light lunch. It's full of subtle flavors that won't
overwhelm your palate, but will make you really happy! The mix of lemony potatoes,
soft butter beans and peppery arugula is a winning combination, especially when served
with juicy vine tomatoes. I love eating this with my Baked Sesame & Tomato Avocados
(page 85), but it also works really well as a side salad, or just on its own with
a good dollop of hummus.

Serves 4

NUT-FREE

¾ pound baby potatoes, well scrubbed

salt and pepper

one 15-ounce can butter beans (or lima
    beans), drained and rinsed

finely grated zest and juice of
    1 unwaxed lemon

olive oil

One 5-ounce package of arugula, or a mix
    of arugula, watercress and spinach

a couple of big vine tomatoes,
    cut into wedges

handful of fresh basil leaves

Put the potatoes into a pan of water, add
a little salt, cover and bring to a boil. Once
boiling, reduce the heat to a simmer and
cook until you can pass a sharp knife through
the middle of the biggest potato. This should
take 10–15 minutes.

Drain the potatoes and put them into a bowl
with the beans, the lemon zest and juice, a
drizzle of olive oil, and salt and pepper to
taste. Mix together and set aside to cool.

Put the salad greens and tomatoes in a
big bowl, season the tomatoes very well,
then scatter the potatoes and beans on top.
Drizzle some olive oil over and top with the
basil to serve.

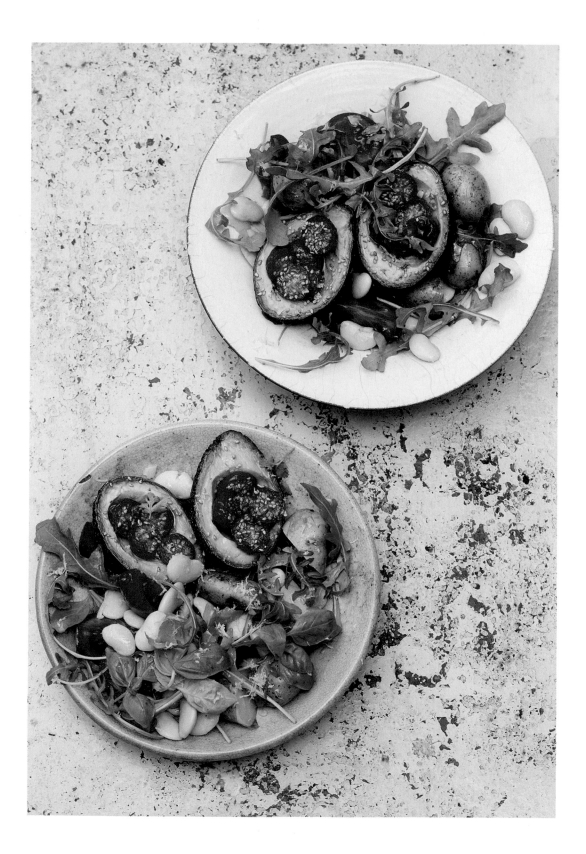

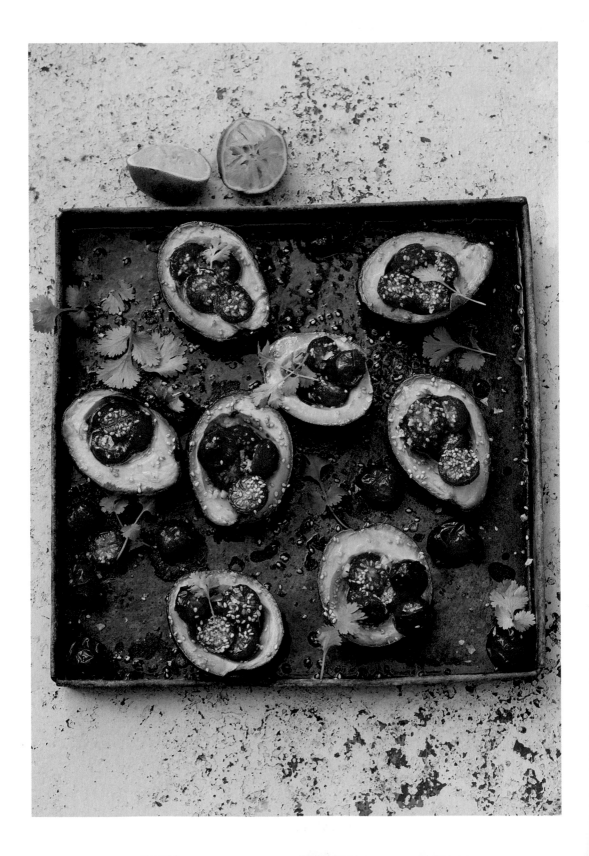

BAKED SESAME & TOMATO AVOCADOS

These taste amazing. If you've never baked an avocado before, you've been missing out!
As the avocado bakes, the tomatoes split open, which makes them extra soft and tender,
while filling them with flavor. They look so beautiful too, with the mix of green and red.
These are a great quick lunch with the Lemony Potato & Butter Bean Salad (page 82),
or with Mango & Mushroom Ceviche (page 66), or as a delicious addition to brunch.

Serves 2 as a main, or 4 with another dish

NUT-FREE

2 avocados

¾ cup cherry tomatoes, plus more if you
  have them

2 garlic cloves, crushed

3 teaspoons sesame oil

olive oil

salt and pepper

4 teaspoons sesame seeds

juice of 2 limes

small handful of cilantro, chopped

Preheat the oven to 400°F.

Halve the avocados and remove the pits.
With a spoon, scoop out a little of the flesh
to make the hole a bit bigger (you don't need
this spare flesh, so now is a good time to
snack on the leftovers).

Cut the tomatoes in half, then mix with the
garlic, 1 teaspoon of the sesame oil, a drizzle
of olive oil and lots of salt and pepper.

Place the avocado halves on a baking
sheet, scrunching up a little foil and resting
each half on top to keep them steady while
they're cooking. Evenly fill them with the
tomato mixture.

Place any spare tomatoes around the
avocados to bake alongside (they look
particularly beautiful if they're on the vine).

Drizzle everything with a little more olive oil,
sprinkle with salt and pepper, then bake for
15–20 minutes.

Put the baked avocados on plates, then
sprinkle 1 teaspoon of the sesame seeds
and squeeze the juice of ½ lime over each
avocado half. Drizzle each with ½ teaspoon
sesame oil. Then scatter over the chopped
cilantro and a little extra salt and serve.

SWEET POTATO NOODLES WITH A CREAMY PEANUT SATAY SAUCE

These noodles were quite a revelation to me. They're so much heartier and more filling than zucchini noodles, and this satay sauce really brings them to life. It's so incredibly creamy, with subtle hints of chile and tangy lime. Together they make for the best pick-me-up dinner, healthy but comforting and bursting with flavor. You will need a spiralizer for this recipe.

Serves 2

FOR THE SAUCE

3 tablespoons crunchy peanut butter
   (or almond butter also works)
5 tablespoons almond milk, plus more if
   needed
1 teaspoon tamari
1 teaspoon chili flakes
juice of 1 lime
1 teaspoon honey
a little olive oil, if needed

FOR THE NOODLES

olive oil
1 celery stalk, finely chopped
5 garlic cloves, crushed
1 inch fresh ginger, finely grated
pinch of salt
9 ounces mushrooms, thinly sliced
2 small sweet potatoes, about 7 ounces
   each, peeled and spiralized
3½ cups baby spinach

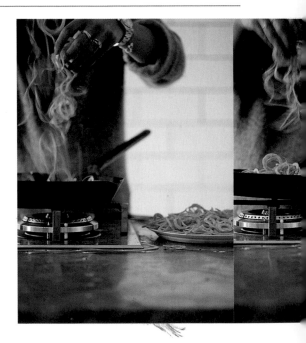

Make the satay sauce. Simply place all the ingredients in a blender and blend until smooth, adding oil if it helps to process the sauce. Add salt to taste.

Heat 1 tablespoon of the oil in a large frying pan, then add the celery, garlic, ginger and salt and sauté over low heat until the celery is softening. Add the mushrooms once the pan has been bubbling for a couple of minutes.

After a minute or so more, add the sweet potatoes and cook for about 10 minutes.

Once the noodles and mushrooms are tender, add the spinach and the satay sauce. Stir until the spinach has wilted and the sauce is warm. If the sauce feels a little thick, add a splash of water, olive oil or almond milk and stir it in until it reaches your desired consistency.

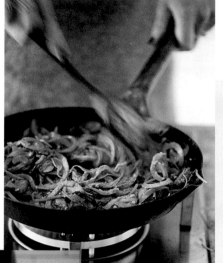

CLEVER COOKING
Slice the ends off the sweet potatoes to create flat surfaces at either end before spiralizing; it makes the process so much easier!

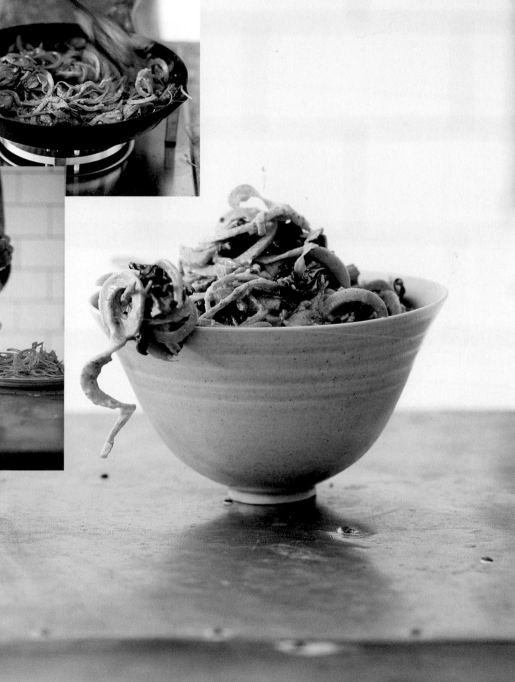

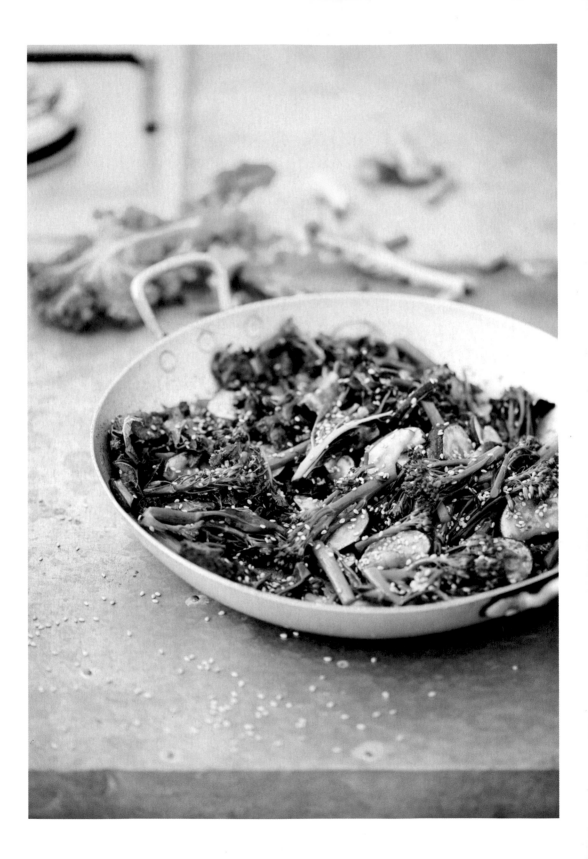

SAUTÉED TAMARI GREENS

These are such a flavorful but incredibly simple way to add goodness to your meal and work perfectly with the Sweet Potato Noodles with a Creamy Peanut Satay Sauce (page 86). The zucchini, broccolini and kale are lightly sautéed in a mix of tamari and sesame oil; a quick way to transform them into something very delicious!

Serves 4

NUT-FREE

3 tablespoons tamari

2 teaspoons sesame oil

1 tablespoon olive oil

2 zucchini, halved lengthwise,
    then cut into half-moons

7 ounces broccolini, each cut into thirds

3½ cups torn-up kale, coarse ribs removed

handful of toasted sesame seeds

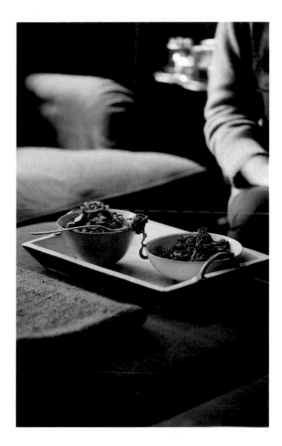

Heat the tamari and oils in a large sauté pan, then add the zucchini and broccolini and stir-fry over high heat for 3 minutes.

Add the kale and cook for another 2 minutes, until the leaves have wilted. Remove from the heat and place on a serving plate.

Scatter with the toasted sesame seeds and bring to the table.

SUPER SPEEDY

10 minutes

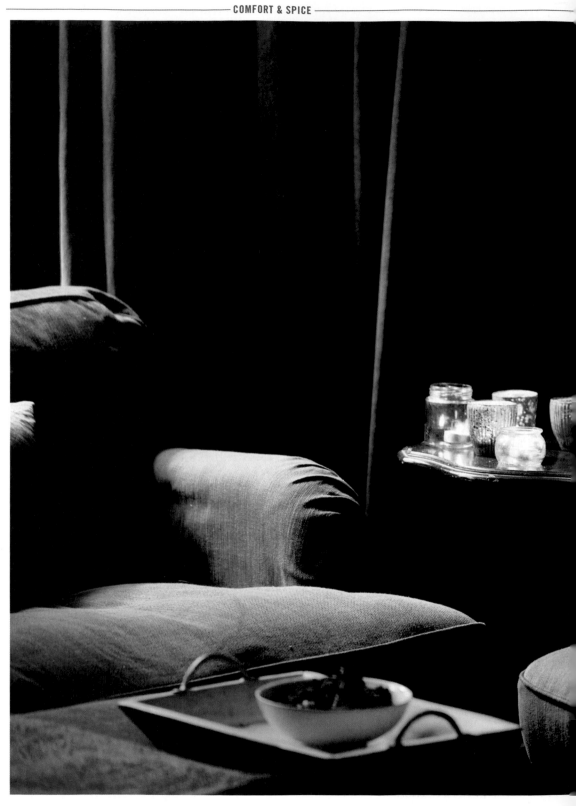

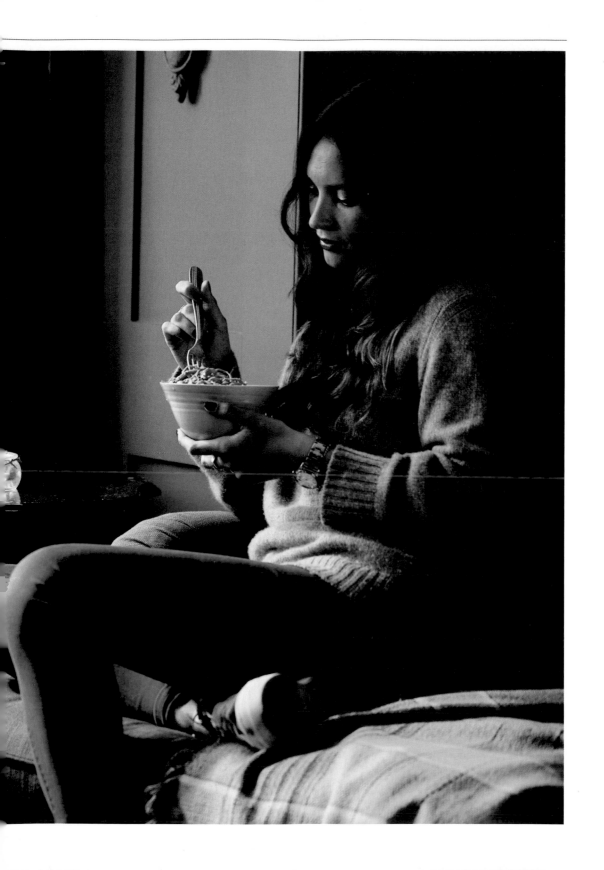

CHILE & GINGER PHO

This is a simplified version of the classic pho recipe, which means you can have dinner on the table in twenty minutes rather than leaving it to simmer for hours! The broth base is flavored with sesame, ginger, green onions, chile and lime and then filled with lots of veggies and buckwheat noodles before being topped with cilantro. A perfect cozy, comforting supper that will warm and rejuvenate you.

Serves 4

NUT-FREE

2 portions of buckwheat noodles
   (or even zucchini noodles)
1 ounce dried shiitake mushrooms
2 teaspoons sesame oil
generous thumb of fresh ginger, finely
   grated
2 garlic cloves, finely grated
2 fresh red chiles, finely sliced
2 green onions, each chopped into quarters
2 tablespoons brown miso paste
2 tablespoons tamari
scant ½ cup baby corn
½ pound bok choy, thinly sliced
1 generous cup bean sprouts
2 carrots, peeled and julienned
handful of cilantro, roughly chopped
juice of 1 lime, plus lime wedges to serve

Prepare the noodles, if using, according to the package instructions, then drain in a sieve and rinse with cold water. Put the dried shiitake in a bowl, pour over 2 cups boiling water and set aside for 20 minutes.

Heat the sesame oil in a wok or large sauté pan. Add the ginger, garlic, chiles and green onions and cook for a minute or so, stirring to make sure the garlic doesn't burn.

Splash in a little water and let it bubble for a couple of minutes, then add the miso and tamari and 2 cups more boiling water. Let this broth bubble away until the mushrooms are ready, then add them too, with their soaking water (except the dregs, as they may contain grit). Return to a nice simmer for 5 minutes.

Add the corn and bok choy, and simmer for 5 minutes. Stir in the bean sprouts and carrots.

Divide the noodles among 4 bowls, then spoon the broth on top. Sprinkle with chopped cilantro and a squeeze of lime juice, then serve with lime wedges.

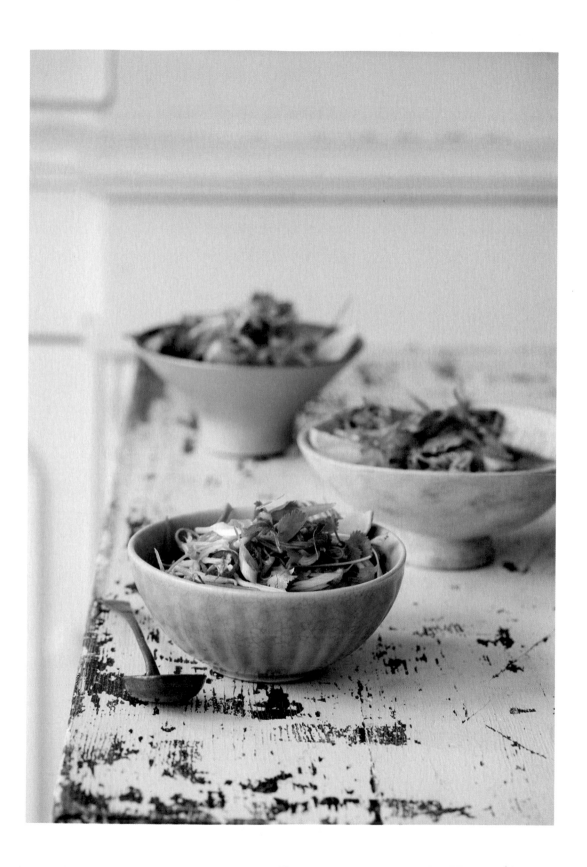

SESAME & MAPLE SUMMER ROLLS WITH SWEET ALMOND DIPPING SAUCE

One of my favorite quick bites. These take just five minutes to make, there's no cooking required and almost no cleanup either, which I love! I serve them to friends when they arrive, as a predinner snack, or use them as a nibble at a party. The flavors work so well with the Chile & Ginger Pho, too (page 92). It's a perfectly light but incredibly delicious meal.

Makes 10

FOR THE ROLLS

1 cucumber, peeled
small handful of cilantro
. juice of 1–2 limes (depending how juicy they are; if you don't get much juice from the first, add the second to get a good lime flavor in the dressing)
1 tablespoon maple syrup
1 tablespoon sesame oil
1 tablespoon sesame seeds
1 tablespoon olive oil
salt
10 rice paper wrappers
1 large avocado, chopped

FOR THE DIPPING SAUCE

1 tablespoon almond butter
1 tablespoon sesame seeds
1 tablespoon olive oil
1 tablespoon sesame oil
1 tablespoon maple syrup
juice of 1 lime
1 tablespoon tamari

Chop the cucumber into thin quarter-rounds and finely chop the cilantro.

Toss the cucumber in a bowl with the cilantro, lime juice, maple syrup, sesame oil and seeds, olive oil and salt to taste and let them all sit in the bowl for a few minutes to marinate.

Get the wrappers ready by dipping each into warm water to soften them. Scoop some of the cucumber mix into the middle of each, then add some avocado. Roll the wrapper up. Repeat to make 10 rolls.

Stir all the sauce ingredients together in a bowl, ready for dipping.

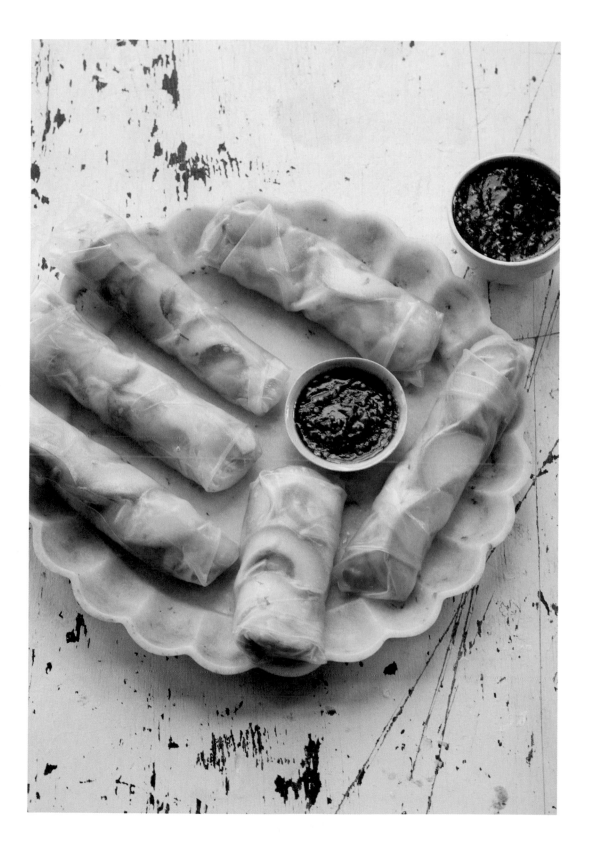

PISTACHIO & APRICOT QUINOA

Wonderfully quick and simple to throw together. This tastes amazing with the soft Asian Sesame Slaw (page 99); together, they're one of my favorite summer lunches. The flavors in this quinoa mixture are wonderfully subtle. The apricots add a lovely sweet, chewy touch, while the bites of cucumber give a freshness and the pistachios create a nutty crunch.

Serves 3

FOR THE QUINOA

1 cup quinoa

salt

1 small cucumber

15 dried apricots (preferably unsulphured)

⅔ cup pistachios

handful of arugula (optional)

FOR THE DRESSING

finely grated zest and juice of
    1 unwaxed lemon

1 teaspoon ground cumin

2 tablespoons apple cider vinegar

4 tablespoons olive oil

salt

Place the quinoa in a saucepan with a generous sprinkling of salt and 2 cups boiling water. Bring to a boil, then let it simmer for 10–15 minutes, until the water has been absorbed and the quinoa is soft and fluffy. Place in a salad bowl and let cool.

Meanwhile, finely chop the cucumber and cut each apricot into 6 pieces.

Mix all the dressing ingredients together.

Mix the cooled quinoa with the cucumber, apricots and most of the pistachios. Then add the dressing and mix it all together.

Finally, sprinkle the remaining pistachios on the top. Serve with arugula, if you like.

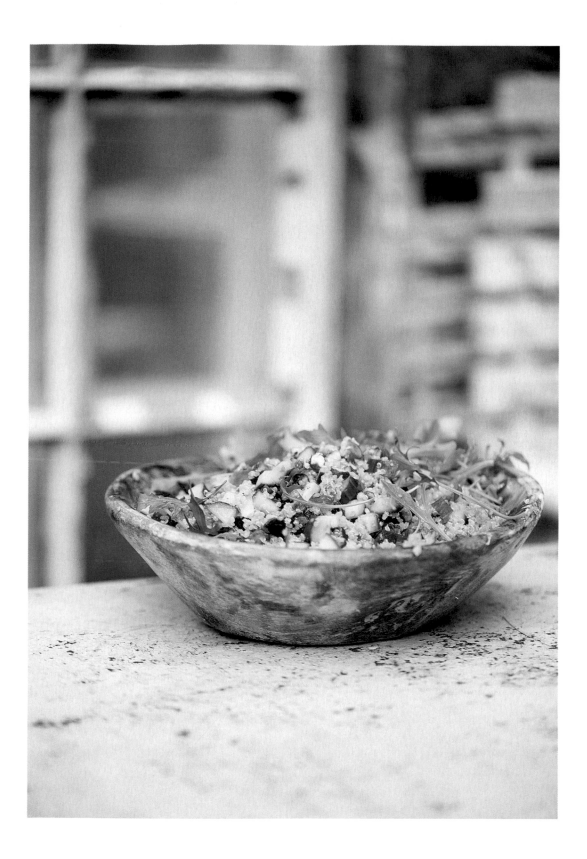

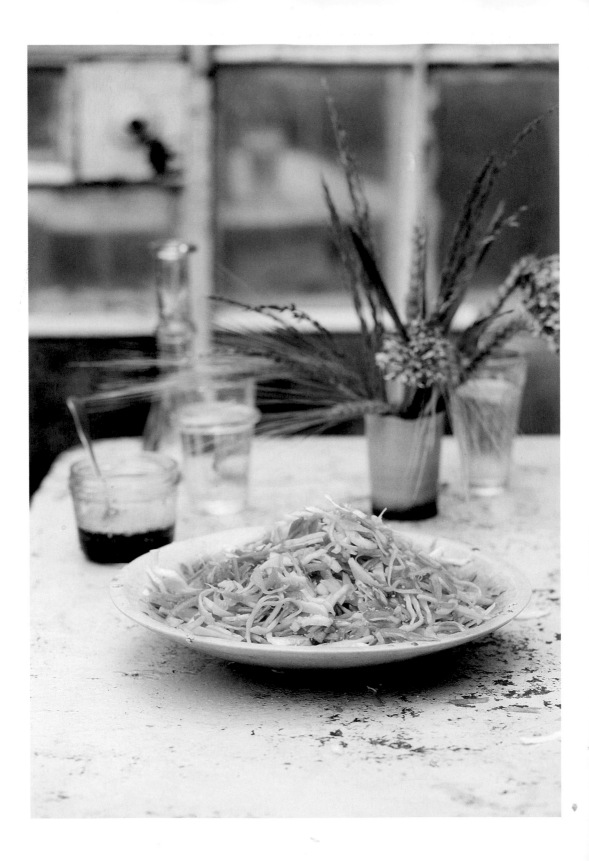

SESAME SLAW

One of my go-to quick salads, this is so easy to make and full of flavor. I know slaw doesn't sound overly exciting—and lots of people wouldn't count cabbage as one of their favorite foods—but this really is so great and so worth trying. I promise you'll be surprised at how much you love it! It tastes amazing with Pistachio & Apricot Quinoa, but I also love it with the Baked Plantains with Sweet Chile Sauce (pages 96 and 187); they are incredible together.

Serves 3

NUT-FREE

2 carrots

⅓ green cabbage

finely grated zest of 1 unwaxed lime
    and juice of 2 limes

2 tablespoons sesame seeds

2 tablespoons sesame oil

5 tablespoons olive oil

2 tablespoons tamari

1 tablespoon honey

generous sprinkling of salt

Start by peeling and grating the carrots (use the fattest holes on the grater, or the grater setting on your food processor). Next, finely shred the cabbage by slicing finely with a sharp knife. Mix together in a bowl.

Add the lime zest and juice to the bowl. Add the sesame seeds, sesame oil, olive oil, tamari, honey and salt and stir well, until the carrots and cabbage are totally covered in dressing.

Let the slaw sit for 10–20 minutes before serving; this allows it to soften and absorb the flavors of the dressing.

SUPER SPEEDY

10 minutes, plus marinating time

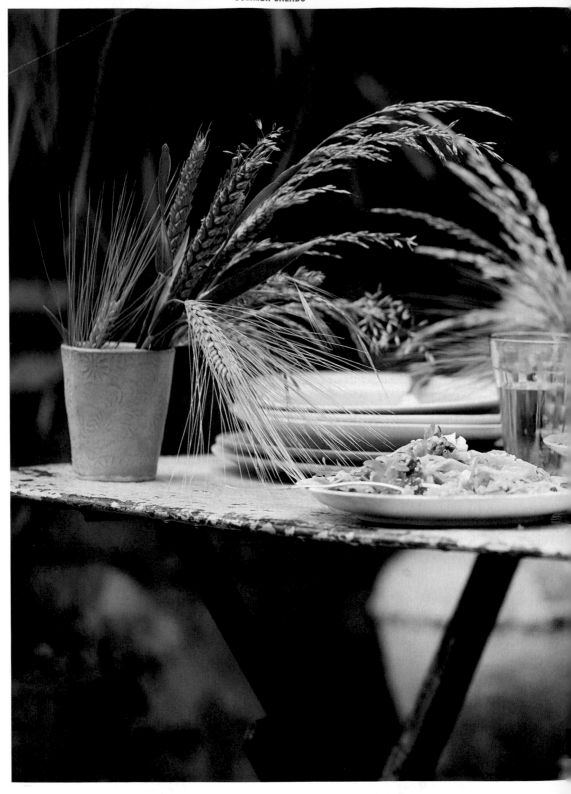

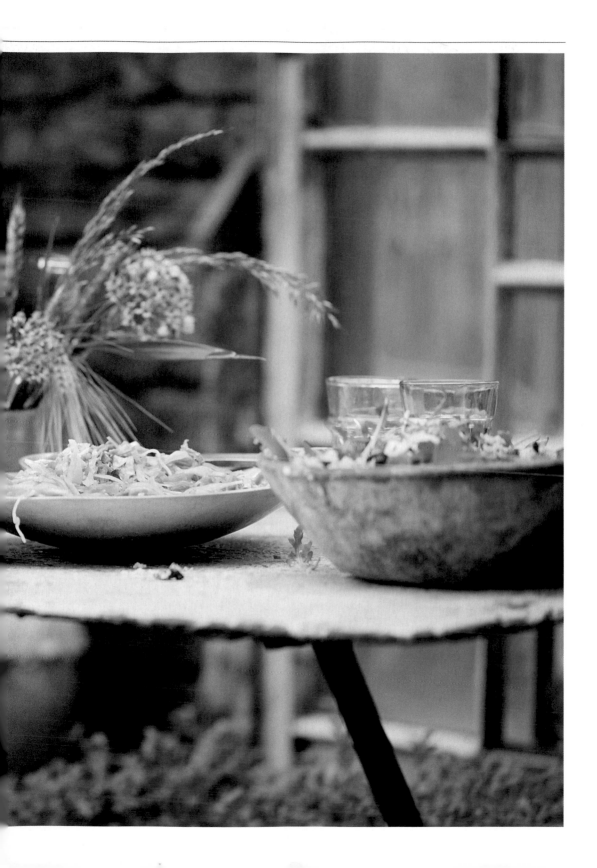

SAUTÉED TEMPEH WITH ROASTED GARLIC & ALMOND PESTO

I've grown to really enjoy tempeh over the last year. It's not overly exciting on its own, but when you sauté it with green onions and tamari, dunk it into a big bowl of roasted garlic and almond pesto and then scatter it across a Sesame, Cilantro & Roasted Fennel Rice Bowl (page 104) it tastes pretty wonderful!

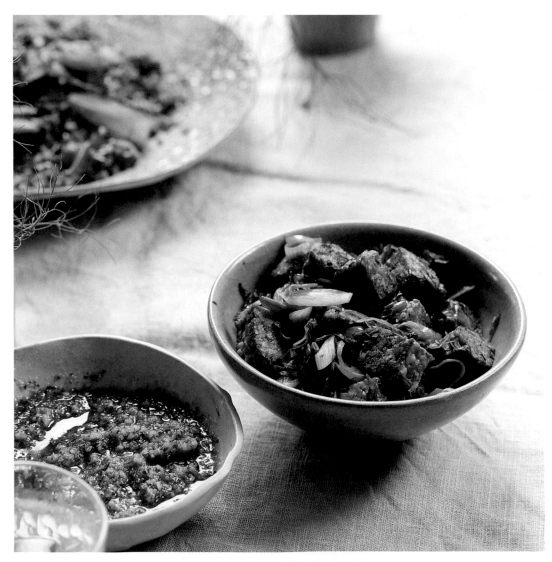

Serves 2

FOR THE PESTO
6 large garlic cloves, unpeeled
scant ¾ cup blanched almonds
2 cups fresh basil leaves
juice of 1 large lemon
½ cup plus 2 tablespoons olive oil
salt

FOR THE TEMPEH
7 ounces tempeh
2 green onions
2 teaspoons coconut oil
1 teaspoon apple cider vinegar
1 teaspoon tamari

For the pesto, preheat the oven to 400°F. Place the garlic and almonds on a baking sheet and bake for 10 minutes, then remove from the oven and let cool.

Once cool, peel the garlic and add it and all the remaining pesto ingredients to a food processor. Blend until smooth. Scrape into a bowl and set aside.

Cut the tempeh into bite-size squares and slice the green onions.

Heat the coconut oil in a frying pan over high heat. Once it has melted, add the green onions, vinegar, tamari and tempeh. Cook for 10 minutes, or until the tempeh browns and turns crispy.

Serve the tempeh on top of the Sesame, Cilantro & Roasted Fennel Rice Bowl with the pesto. Or add it to any other bowl. I find it's best alongside some quinoa or brown rice.

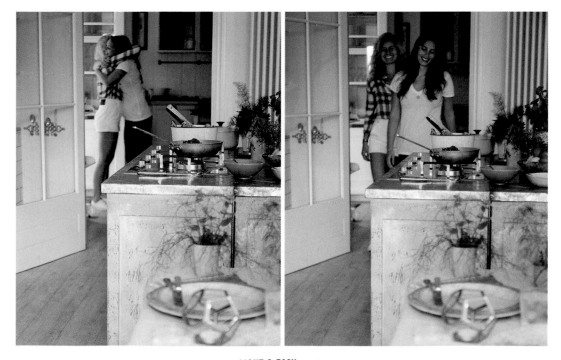

SESAME, CILANTRO & ROASTED
FENNEL RICE BOWL

This brown rice bowl with creamy avocado chunks, blackened peppers, roasted fennel
and mashed garlic dressing is incredible, one of my absolute best dinners. It's great just
on its own, but I also love serving it in bowls with sautéed tempeh scattered over the
top and a big dollop of creamy Roasted Garlic & Almond Pesto on the side (page 102),
which I then dip each bite into for extra flavor!

Serves 2

NUT-FREE

FOR THE RICE BOWL

⅓ cup short-grain brown rice

1 tablespoon apple cider vinegar

1 tablespoon tamari

salt

1 fennel bulb

2 red bell peppers

olive oil

2–4 tablespoons cilantro

1 avocado

2 tablespoons sesame seeds

FOR THE DRESSING

4 garlic cloves, unpeeled

3 tablespoons olive oil

2 teaspoons apple cider vinegar

1 teaspoon tamari

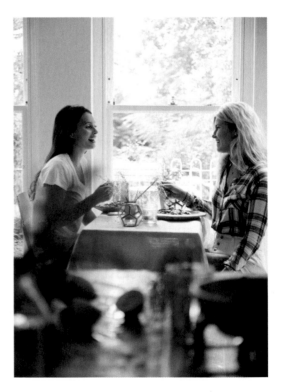

Cook the brown rice in 1 cup water with the vinegar, tamari and salt to taste. This should take about 40 minutes.

Preheat the oven to 400°F.

Slice the fennel lengthwise. Cut each pepper into about 8 pieces. Place them on a baking sheet, drizzle with olive oil and sprinkle with salt. Bake for 15–20 minutes, until the edges are browning. For the last 10 minutes, add the garlic cloves (they will be used in the dressing).

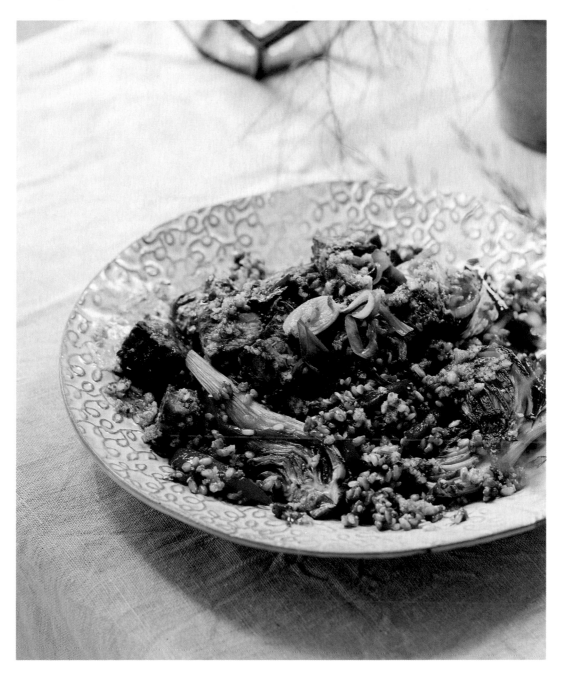

Let the rice, veg and garlic cool.

Finely chop the cilantro. Cut the avocado into bite-size chunks. Roughly chop the roast veg and stir into the rice, with the avocado and sesame seeds.

Make the dressing. Peel the garlic and mash with a fork (it should be really soft). Mix in all the other ingredients. Stir into the rice and sprinkle with the cilantro. Serve in a beautiful salad bowl.

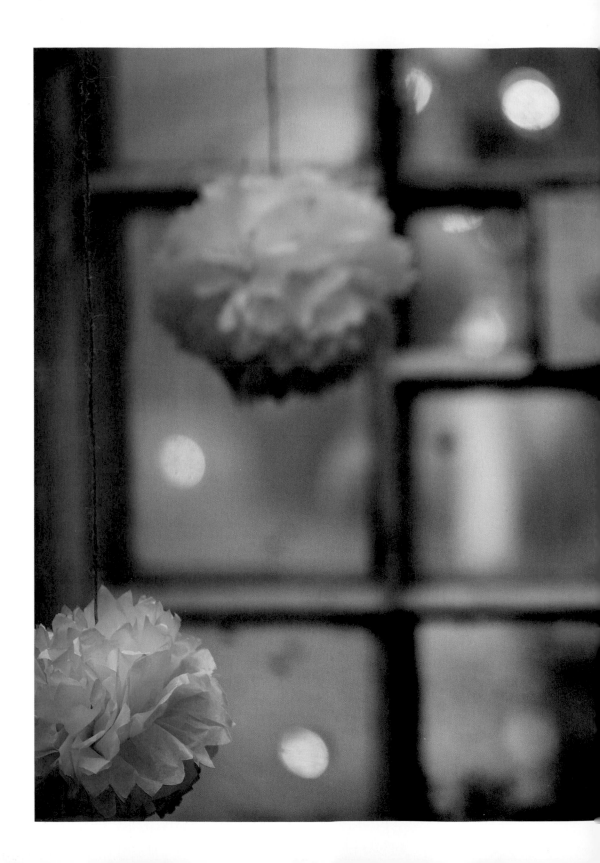

FEASTS

LONG, LAZY DINNERS TO SHARE & SAVOR

FEASTS

*Feasting with friends is one of the best things you can do in life,
almost nothing makes me happier than sharing mountains of beautiful
food with the people I love most, and that's what this chapter is
all about. I hope it will help you find ways to enjoy with others the
kind of food you love, so they'll see how delicious nutritious food can be.
There are so many amazing meals here, but I'm especially keen on bowls
of Pea, Zucchini & Coconut Risotto served with Chile-Garlic Broccoli
for cozy evenings; big platters of Quesadillas with Cashew Sour
Cream & Guacamole, Refried Black Beans & Spicy Salsa for fun nights
with friends; and Marinated Cauliflower Steaks with Chile Quinoa
and Sun-Dried Tomato & Butter Bean Hummus for summer nights.*

MENU

MEXICAN FIESTA

Quesadillas
Refried Black Beans & Spicy Salsa
Cashew Sour Cream & Guacamole

COMFORTING

Pea, Zucchini & Coconut Risotto
Chile-Garlic Broccoli

SUNDAY LUNCH

Herbed Nut Roast
Maple-Roasted Root Veg
Mushroom Gravy

INDIAN FEAST

Chana Masala
Aloo Gobi
Coconut Rice

GARDEN PARTY

Marinated Cauliflower Steaks with Chile Quinoa
Sun-Dried Tomato & Butter Bean Hummus

COZY KITCHEN SUPPER

Three-Bean Stew
Mango Salsa

SIMPLE & INEXPENSIVE

Chickpea Chili in Baked Sweet Potatoes
Spiced Roast Cauliflower

CURRY NIGHT IN

My Favorite Curried Veggies
Lime & Chile Pickle

DATE NIGHT

Tomato & Eggplant Bake
Spinach with Mustard Seeds

QUESADILLAS

This is such a winner; I've always loved quesadillas, so I'm really excited to share this recipe with you. They were my favorite meal and I hadn't had them in so long until I created this. Everyone always adores being served one of these beautiful quesadillas. It's a fun meal, and definitely shows people that healthy eating isn't all about kale and carrots . . . These are best eaten hot and always shared with great friends. They're fun to eat and can get a little messy, so don't make them for a first date!

Makes 4 quesadillas

NUT-FREE

FOR THE TORTILLAS

1⅔ cups buckwheat flour

1½ cups cornmeal

7 tablespoons ground chia seeds

2 teaspoons salt

olive oil

FOR THE QUESADILLAS

Refried Black Beans & Spicy Salsa (page 113)

Cashew Sour Cream & Guacamole (page 115)

Preheat the oven to 400°F.

Make the tortillas. Mix all the ingredients except the oil in a bowl, then gradually add 1¼ cups water, mixing it into a paste with a fork.

On a work surface, lay down a square of parchment paper. Cut another square of parchment and set aside.

Wet your hands, pick up one-eighth of the tortilla mixture and roll it into a nice smooth ball. Drop the ball into the center of the parchment, place the second sheet of parchment on top and squash the dough down gently into a disc. With a rolling pin, roll it from the center outward to make a round about 8 inches across, then place on a baking sheet. Leave both sheets of parchment in place. Repeat to make 8 tortillas.

Pop them in the oven for 4 minutes. Peel off the parchment and set the tortillas aside.

Make the quesadillas. Heat a large nonstick frying pan over high heat. Add a little olive oil, place a tortilla in the pan and load it up with the fillings. Place another tortilla on top, press down to flatten, and cook for 2 minutes. Then flip over gently with a spatula and cook for another 1–2 minutes on the second side. Remove from the heat and cut into quarters or eighths. Repeat to make 3 more quesadillas.

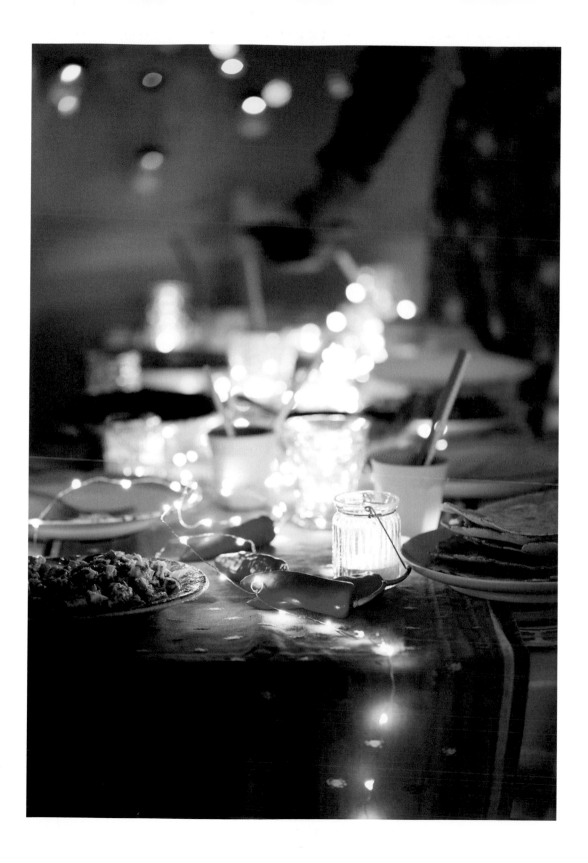

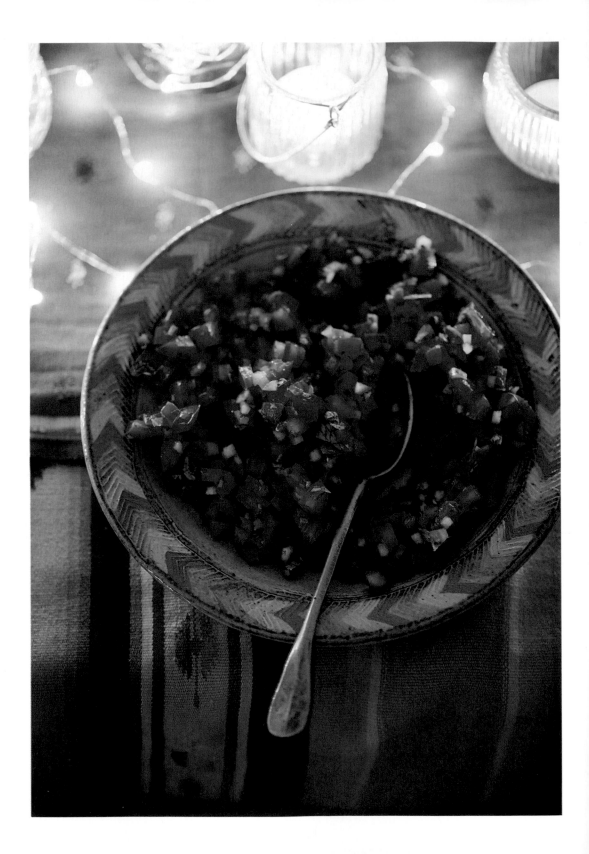

REFRIED BLACK BEANS & SPICY SALSA

These make the most delicious quesadilla filling (page 110). The black beans cook to a comforting, warming mix with a delicious blend of flavors. The tomato salsa brings a slightly spicy and fresher element to the dish, while the beans are heartier with a richer, saltier flavor.

Makes enough for 4 generous quesadillas

NUT-FREE

FOR THE BLACK BEANS

olive oil

4 garlic cloves, crushed

salt and pepper

1 teaspoon ground coriander

½ teaspoon smoked paprika

two 15-ounce cans black beans, drained and rinsed

juice of 1 lime

FOR THE SALSA

5 tomatoes, finely chopped

2 fresh red chiles, seeded and finely chopped

1 tablespoon apple cider vinegar

2 tablespoons olive oil

handful of cilantro, chopped

Start by making the black beans. Heat a glug of olive oil in a saucepan, then add the garlic and salt and pepper to taste and fry over medium heat for about 1 minute until it starts to turn translucent but doesn't color.

Add the spices, beans and lime juice. Cook over low heat for about 10 minutes, or until the beans start to soften.

Meanwhile, for the salsa, mix everything together in a bowl. Cover and let sit for at least 5 minutes before eating, so that all the flavors meld together.

MIX IT UP

I've used 2 chiles in the salsa because I love the spicy heat but, if you prefer, use fewer to your taste.

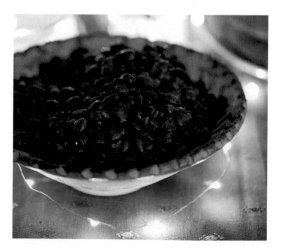

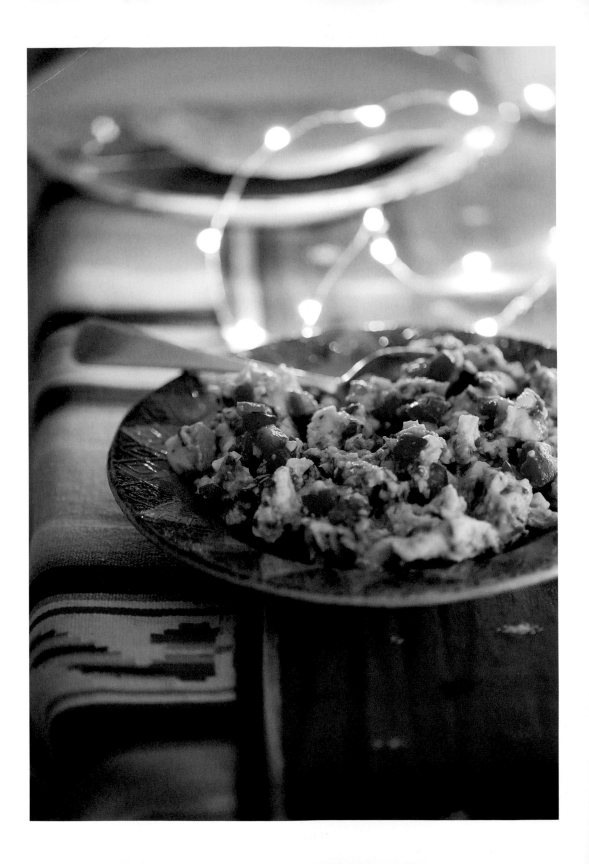

CASHEW SOUR CREAM & GUACAMOLE

These are wonderful additions to quesadillas, as they make each bite so creamy. I originally made the cashew sour cream for my Mini Baked Potatoes (page 210), but it was so good I decided I definitely needed to use it in the quesadillas, too! It has a beautifully smooth texture with wonderful flavors from the chives, vinegar and lemon juice, plus I find it works perfectly in quesadillas with this chunky guacamole. Remember that you need to allow soaking time for the cashews.

Makes enough for 4 quesadillas

FOR THE CASHEW SOUR CREAM
1 cup cashews
juice of 1½ lemons
1 tablespoon apple cider vinegar
salt and pepper
1 tablespoon chopped chives
3 green onions, finely chopped

FOR THE GUACAMOLE
3 avocados
juice of 2 limes
1 fresh chile, seeded and finely chopped
1 tomato, seeded and finely chopped
handful of cilantro, finely chopped

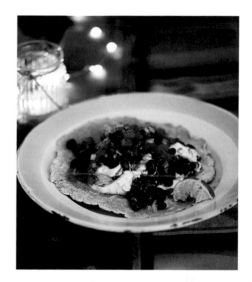

Start the cashew sour cream ahead of time: put the cashews in a bowl, cover with water and let soak for 4 hours.

Drain the cashews and place them in a high-powered blender. Add 2 tablespoons water, the lemon juice, vinegar and salt and pepper to taste. Blend until creamy; this should take a few minutes. Add the chives and green onions and blend for a few seconds, so they are broken down but not blended smooth. If you'd like a thinner consistency, add a little more water.

For the guacamole, scoop the flesh into a bowl. Mash with a fork.

Add the remaining guacamole ingredients and season well.

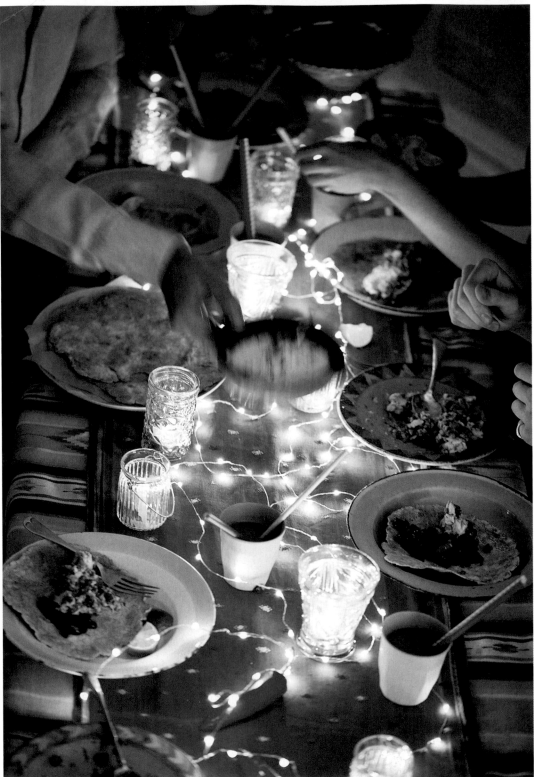

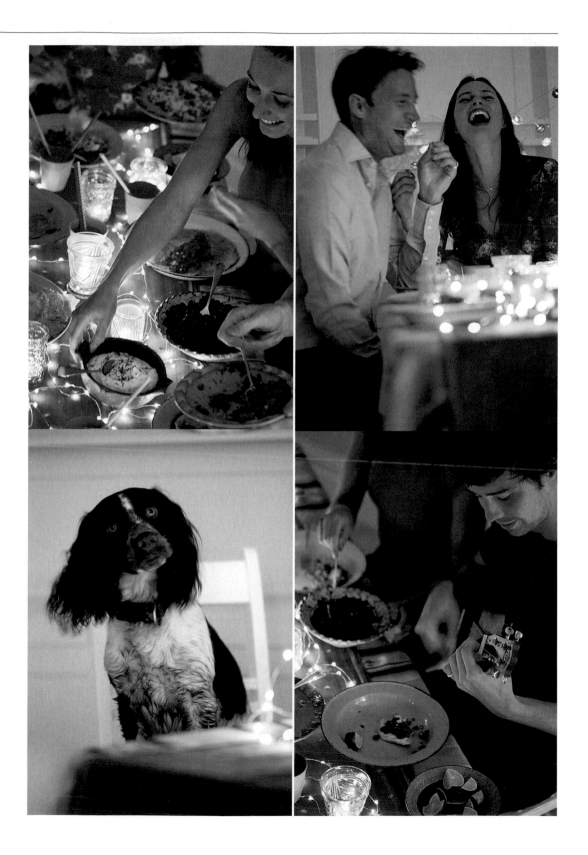

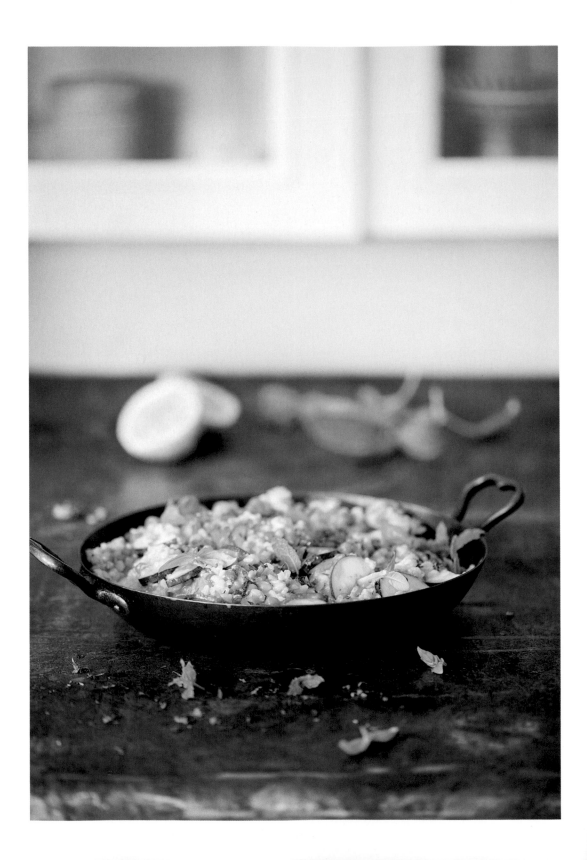

PEA, ZUCCHINI & COCONUT RISOTTO

This is an absolute dream. It's so wonderfully creamy and flavorful, yet still light and refreshing. I cook the rice in coconut milk to give it a more traditional risotto texture, then stir in a creamy blend of puréed peas with lemon juice and olive oil to give the finished dish extra flavor and thickness. The first time I made this I shared it with my sister—who's a risotto addict—and she said that she didn't even need to add parmesan cheese . . . which was the ultimate compliment from her!

Serves 4

FOR THE RISOTTO

olive oil

2 celery stalks, finely chopped

salt and pepper

5 garlic cloves, crushed

1¾ cups short-grain brown rice

one 14-ounce can coconut milk

2 tablespoons apple cider vinegar

juice of 1 lemon

2 small zucchini, sliced into half-moons

2 cups frozen peas, thawed

a few sprigs of fresh mint, leaves picked
  and roughly chopped

FOR THE CREAMY PEA MIXTURE

1½ cups frozen peas, thawed

juice of 2 lemons

½ cup fresh basil leaves

2 tablespoons nutritional yeast

⅓ cup olive oil

salt and pepper

Put a big glug of olive oil in a large saucepan with a lid and set it over medium heat. Add the celery and salt and pepper to taste and cook for about 10 minutes or until soft. Add the garlic and cook for another minute before adding the rice, coconut milk, 5 cups water, the vinegar and lemon juice. Bring to a boil, then reduce the heat, cover and simmer for 50 minutes, or until the rice is cooked and the water is absorbed. Check it every now and again and give it a stir. You may need to add slightly more water during cooking, as the water can be absorbed at different speeds depending on the shape of your pan and the heat under it.

When the 50 minutes are up, uncover, stir in the zucchini and cook for 5 minutes. Throw in the peas, stir again, and cook for another 5 minutes, then remove from the heat.

Meanwhile, make the pea mixture. Place all the ingredients in a blender, season well and blend until smooth.

Stir the creamy pea mixture into the risotto, sprinkle with the chopped mint and serve.

CHILE-GARLIC BROCCOLI

This is a wonderfully simple side that goes with absolutely everything, though I find it especially good with the Pea, Zucchini & Coconut Risotto (page 119). I love the contrast of the slightly crunchy broccolini and the soft, creamy risotto. It's a lovely way to up the amount of greens in any meal, while adding more flavor and extra texture. I normally use at least six cloves of sautéed garlic in this as I like the flavor to be really strong and come through in every bite, but feel free to tone it down if you want something equally delicious but more subtle.

Serves 4 as a side dish

NUT-FREE

olive oil

4–6 garlic cloves, crushed

1 fresh red chile, seeded and finely chopped

salt and pepper

14 ounces broccolini, trimmed and cut
   into thirds

juice of ½ lemon

Heat a good glug of olive oil in a wok or a large saucepan over medium heat. Add the garlic, chile and salt and pepper to taste. Cook about 3 minutes, or until the garlic has softened but not colored.

Add the broccolini to the pan, increase the heat, add the lemon juice and—while keeping it moving using a wooden spoon—cook for about 5 minutes, or until it's tender on the outside but still with a little bite.

SUPER SPEEDY

10 minutes

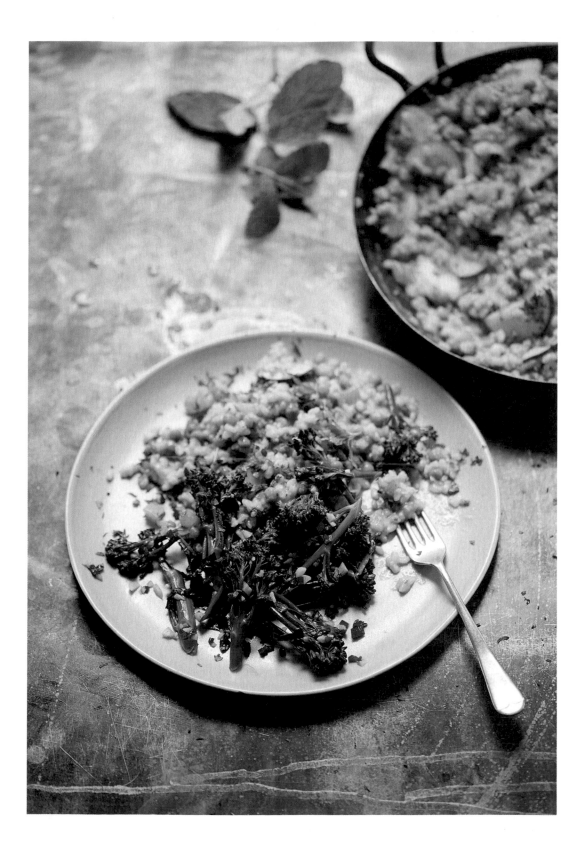

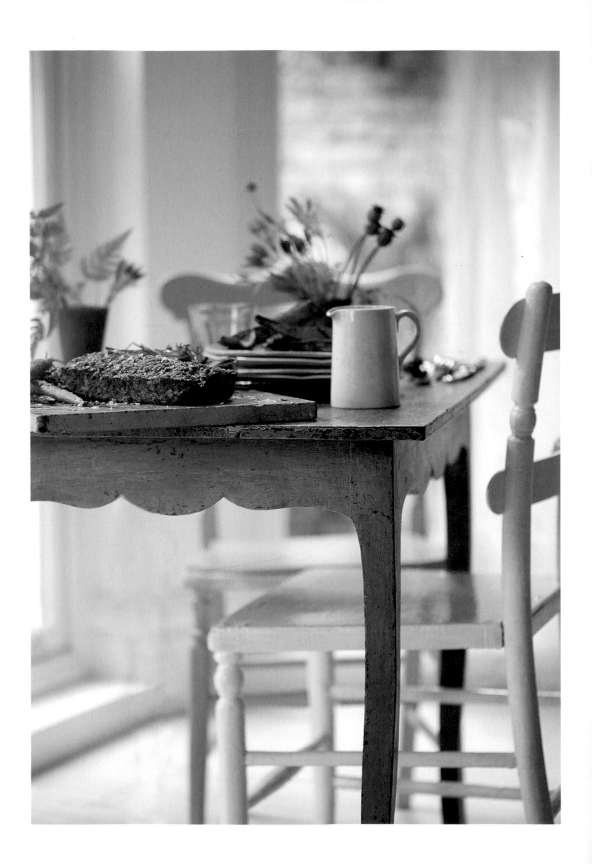

HERBED NUT ROAST

This is the ideal veggie option to share with friends for a long, lazy Sunday lunch. It's lovely and hearty and full of flavor from the pine nuts and cashews to the nutmeg, garlic, sage, tarragon, garlic and parsley. I love this with a pile of Maple-Roasted Root Veg and a big spoonful of Smashed Turmeric & Mustard Seed Potatoes (pages 126 and 180).

Serves 6

2 tablespoons olive oil, plus more for the pan

6 tablespoons pine nuts

generous ½ cup cashews

1 celery stalk, finely chopped

7 ounces butternut squash, peeled and finely chopped

1 medium carrot, peeled and finely chopped

salt and pepper

3 garlic cloves, crushed

5 ounces cremini mushrooms, finely chopped

2 fresh sage leaves, roughly chopped

1 tablespoon roughly chopped fresh parsley

1 tablespoon roughly chopped fresh tarragon

a few good gratings of nutmeg

5 tablespoons rolled oats

½ cup plus 1 tablespoon brown rice flour

½ tablespoon ground chia seeds

Mushroom Gravy (page 126)

CLEVER COOKING

You need roughly the top part of a butternut squash for this (the bit from the stem end to the bulge), so save the rest for later or use it as a side, roasted or mashed. Also, you can roast the squash seeds with a drizzle of oil and seasoning for 10 minutes, then sprinkle them over sautéed greens.

Preheat the oven to 400°F. Oil a 9 x 5-inch loaf pan or line it with parchment paper. Place the pine nuts and cashews on a baking sheet and roast them in the oven for about 10 minutes. They should look golden and give off a toasty aroma when you take them out. Set aside to cool.

Meanwhile, place a large nonstick pan over medium heat and heat the 2 tablespoons oil. Saute the celery, squash and carrot in the oil with lots of salt and pepper. When the celery has started to turn translucent, add the garlic and cook for 1 minute. Add the mushrooms and cook for 5 minutes. Finally, add the herbs and nutmeg and stir well.

Place half the nuts in a food processor with the oats and whizz up as fine as they will go. Coarsely chop the remaining nuts, so they aren't too chunky, then add these and the ground nut mixture to the pan. Add the flour and chia seeds and mix well.

Press into the prepared loaf pan, cover with foil and bake for 35 minutes. Take the foil off and bake for another 15 minutes. Let cool in the pan on a cooling rack for 15 minutes (it will still be nice and hot). Take it out of the pan and cut into slices; be gentle, as it can crumble. Prepare and serve with Mushroom Gravy.

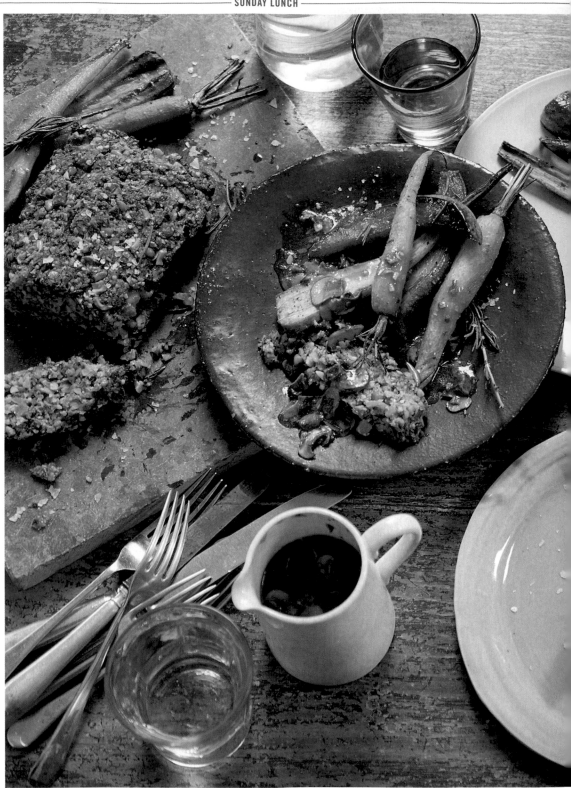

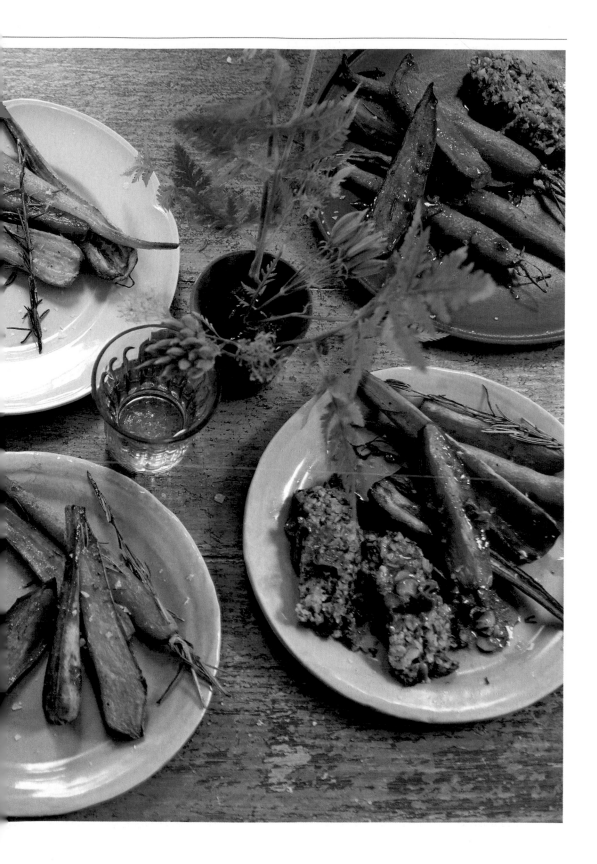

MAPLE-ROASTED ROOT VEG

*A really simple recipe, but the best addition to your Sunday lunch. Maple syrup brings
out the natural sweetness of the veggies, while the paprika, cayenne and rosemary add
a whole new level of flavor. The veg become so sweet and tender when baked like this,
so everyone will love them! If you're not ready to go full veggie and serve these with a
nut loaf, then try adding them to a conventional roast instead; it's a great way to start
getting your friends and family excited about plant-based meals.*

Serves 4–6

NUT-FREE

2 sweet potatoes, scrubbed well
4 carrots, peeled
4 parsnips, peeled
olive oil
3 tablespoons maple syrup
1 teaspoon smoked paprika
½ teaspoon cayenne pepper
6 sprigs of fresh rosemary
salt and pepper

Preheat the oven to 400°F.

Cut the sweet potatoes into equal-size wedges
and halve the carrots and parsnips lengthwise.
Place on a large baking sheet in a single layer,
or spread them over 2 sheets. Drizzle with
olive oil and the maple syrup, then sprinkle
the paprika and cayenne over. Toss everything
together, then tuck the rosemary into the veg
and season with salt and pepper to taste.

Roast for 1 hour, turning once or twice in that
time. When they're finished cooking, the veg
should be golden and sticky, with edges that
are slightly crisp . . . delicious!

MUSHROOM GRAVY

*The mushrooms and tamari give deeply savory flavors to this gravy. Sharpened with a
little mustard and made aromatic with tarragon, it makes Sunday lunch a real treat.
This makes enough for the Herbed Nut Roast (page 123), but if you like lots
of gravy, double the quantities here.*

Makes enough for the nut roast

0.4 ounce dried porcini mushrooms
2 tablespoons canola oil, more if needed
5 ounces cremini mushrooms, thinly sliced
2 garlic cloves, crushed

salt and pepper
1 tablespoon finely chopped fresh tarragon
1 teaspoon Dijon mustard
1 tablespoon cornstarch
1 tablespoon tamari

the pan is dry, add a bit more oil.) Keep the garlic moving so it doesn't brown, or it will be bitter. Scoop the porcini out of the water, finely chop and add to the pan, reserving the soaking liquid.

Once the garlic is translucent, add the tarragon, 1⅔ cups mushroom soaking liquid (avoiding any grit from the bottom of the bowl) and the mustard. Mix the cornstarch with 1 tablespoon water to a paste, add to the pan and let simmer for 5–10 minutes, until it has a nice consistency. Stir in the tamari.

Put the dried porcini in a bowl with 2 cups boiling water and soak for at least 10 minutes.

Heat the oil in a nonstick frying pan over high heat. Add the fresh mushrooms and let them color on both sides, then reduce the heat to low, add the garlic and season. (If

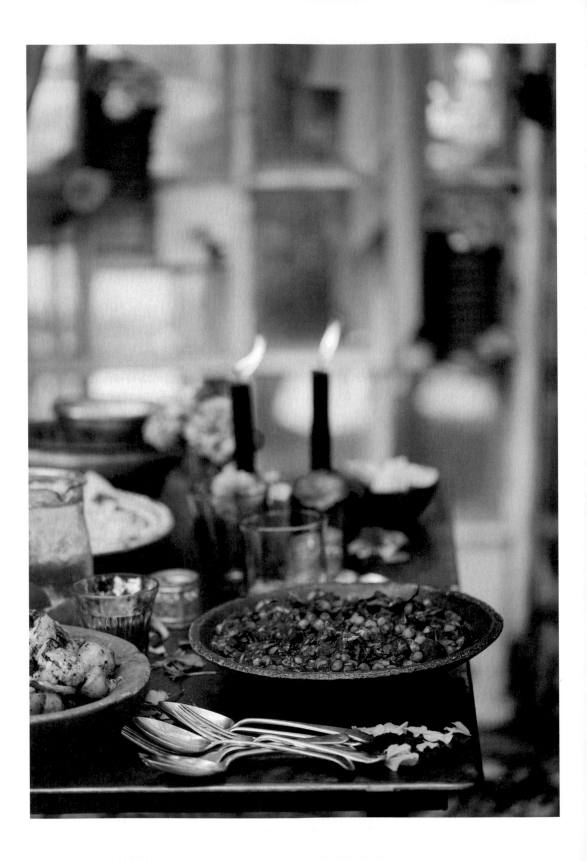

CHANA MASALA

*Absolutely delicious and filled with incredible spices that really transform the chickpeas.
I also add leeks and spinach, as I love getting the extra veg in and they add a great
flavor, plus the green of the spinach makes the meal look beautiful, too. I love this served
alongside my Aloo Gobi and Coconut Rice (pages 130 and 133), with a generous dollop
of coconut yogurt.*

Serves 6

NUT-FREE

5 tablespoons olive oil

6 curry leaves, or 1 teaspoon curry powder

1 leek, finely chopped

½ teaspoon ground turmeric

2 tablespoons ground cumin

2 tablespoons ground coriander

2 tablespoons garam masala

1 teaspoon chili powder

1 onion, finely chopped

1 inch fresh ginger, finely grated

5 garlic cloves, finely grated

two 14.5-ounce cans diced tomatoes

2 tablespoons tomato paste

2 fresh green finger chiles, halved
   lengthwise

salt and pepper

two 15-ounce cans chickpeas,
   drained and rinsed

9 ounces baby spinach

juice of ½ lemon

cilantro leaves, to serve

CLEVER COOKING

Make extra so that you have leftovers to
enjoy in your lunch box! As with most curries,
this tastes even better the next day, as the
flavors have had a chance to develop further.

Heat the oil in a large saucepan and throw
in the curry leaves, if using. Let them sizzle
away and release their flavor for a few
minutes, then drop in the leek and stir.

Next add the dry spices—including the curry
powder if you're not using curry leaves—and
stir so that they're mixed nicely with the leek.
Let this cook for a few minutes before adding
the onion, ginger and garlic; at this point you
can add 1–2 tablespoons water if things are
starting to stick to the pan. Cook for a few
minutes before adding the canned tomatoes,
tomato paste, green chiles and plenty of
salt and pepper. After you've poured in
the tomatoes from their cans, swish a little
water around in each to get the remaining
juice, then add this to the saucepan, too. Let
everything bubble away for 20 minutes.

Add the chickpeas and cook for another
10 minutes.

Stir in the spinach, just until it wilts. Let cool
slightly, then stir in the lemon juice and serve
in shallow bowls, sprinkling cilantro leaves
over the curry.

ALOO GOBI

Matt and I have a favorite little Indian restaurant near our flat that we go to all the time, and I always get the aloo gobi and chana masala. I think the two taste so great together and when I make them at home I serve them on a bed of creamy Coconut Rice (page 133), which makes the meal even better. I love the mix of flavors, which transform the cauliflower and potato into something very special that I hope you'll all really enjoy.

Serves 6

NUT-FREE

2 small heads cauliflower, broken into florets
4 tablespoons olive oil
salt and pepper
1 pound baby potatoes, well scrubbed, quartered
½ cinnamon stick
½ teaspoon black peppercorns
5 green cardamom pods, bashed
1 tablespoon mustard seeds
½ teaspoon ground turmeric
2 teaspoons ground cumin
2 teaspoons ground coriander
5 garlic cloves, finely grated
1 inch fresh ginger, finely grated
⅔ cup cherry tomatoes, halved
2 tablespoons tomato paste
1 tablespoon apple cider vinegar
2 green finger chiles, sliced
juice of ½ lemon
cilantro leaves, chopped, to serve

Preheat the oven to 425°F.

Place the cauliflower on a large rimmed baking sheet, drizzle with a little of the oil, sprinkle with salt and roast for 20 minutes, giving it a shake halfway through cooking.

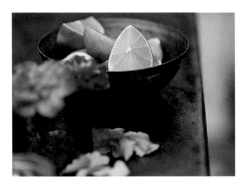

Meanwhile, in a saucepan of boiling water, cook the potatoes for 10–15 minutes, until tender. Drain and set aside.

Gently heat the remaining olive oil in a large saucepan. Add all the dry spices. Cook for a few minutes, stirring every now and again, until you start to smell the aromas being released.

Now add the garlic, ginger, tomatoes, tomato paste, vinegar and green chiles, pour in a scant 1 cup water and cook for about 3 minutes. Add the cooked potatoes and cauliflower, squeeze on the lemon juice, season generously with salt and pepper and stir so that all the vegetables are coated in the spiced sauce.

Cook for 5 minutes, then it's ready to eat.

Sprinkle with the cilantro and eat with Chana Masala and Coconut Rice (pages 129 and 133).

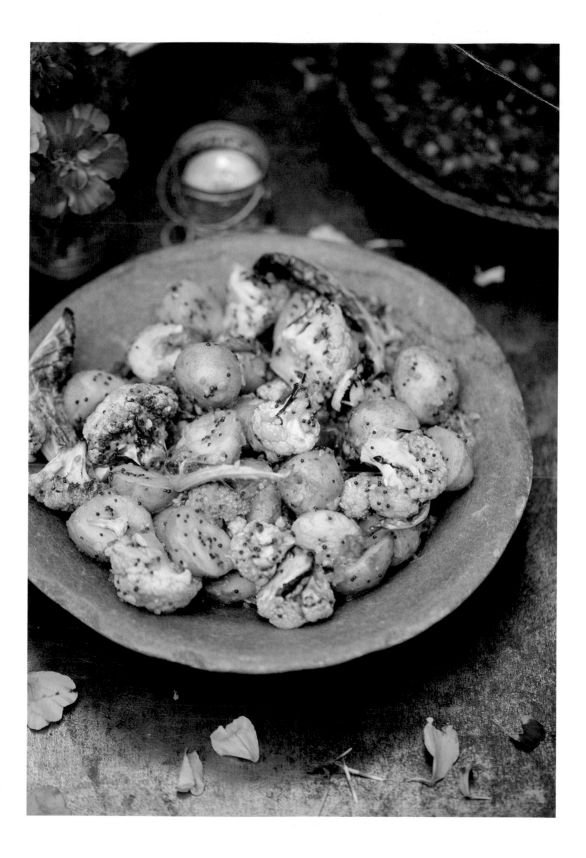

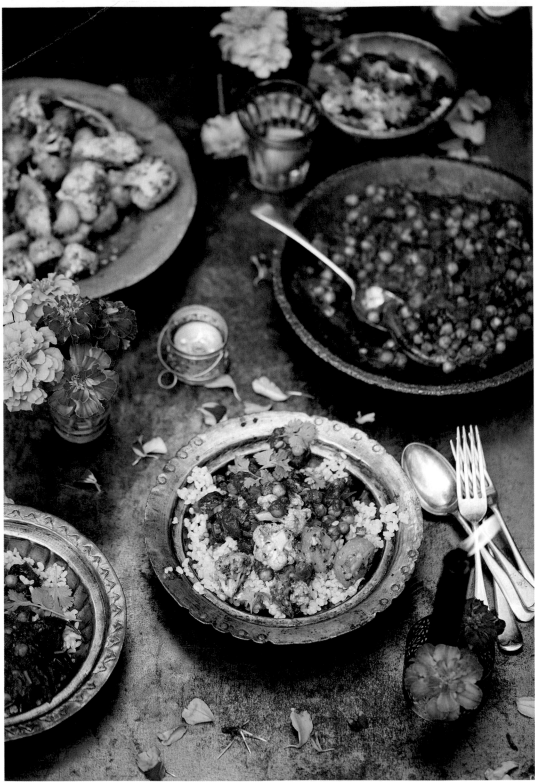

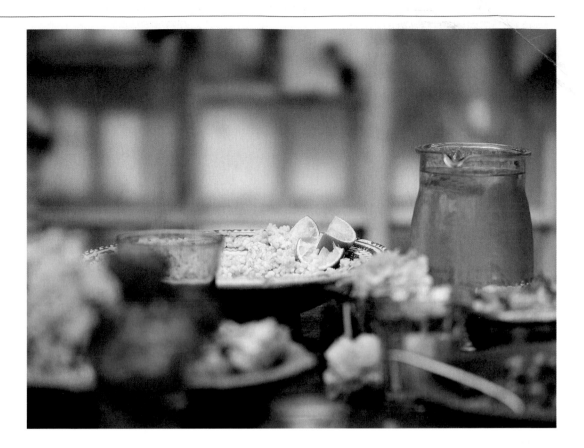

COCONUT RICE

I first ate coconut rice on a trip to Colombia a few years ago and really fell in love with it; it's the best way to make humble rice into something really fabulous. I think it makes the perfect base for your Indian-inspired feast, as it's subtle and simple, which means it's able to soak up all the incredible flavors and spices of the Aloo Gobi and Chana Masala (pages 130 and 129), while adding its own creamy element to each bite.

Serves 6

2½ cups short-grain brown rice
one 14-ounce can coconut milk
juice of 2 limes
salt

Put the rice, coconut milk, lime juice, generous sprinkling of salt and 3¾ cups boiling water in a pan. Stir well and cover the pan.

Bring to a boil, then reduce the heat to a simmer and cook for about 45 minutes, or until all liquid has evaporated.

CLEVER COOKING
Try making your rice like this to serve with all your stews and curries. Your friends will love it!

MARINATED CAULIFLOWER STEAKS WITH CHILE QUINOA

This dish is just bursting with flavor. The cauliflower steaks are marinated for an hour in a beautiful mix of spices and lemon juice, then baked to create something really special. I serve them on a bed of avocado- and spinach-filled quinoa infused with cilantro, sesame oil and tamari. It all sounds, looks and tastes so impressive, but don't worry, it's actually a really easy meal to pull off! Make sure you add Sun-Dried Tomato & Butter Bean Hummus on the side (page 137), as it really finishes the dish off perfectly.

Serves 4

NUT-FREE

FOR THE CAULIFLOWER STEAKS

2 heads cauliflower, cut from top to base into four 1-inch-thick "steaks"

2 teaspoons ground cumin

2 teaspoons paprika

½ teaspoon chili powder

½ teaspoon ground turmeric

3½ tablespoons olive oil

juice of ½ lemon

salt and pepper

FOR THE CHILE QUINOA

1¼ cups quinoa

½ cup cilantro, finely chopped

1 fresh red chile, seeded and finely chopped

1 avocado

3 tablespoons olive oil

2 tablespoons apple cider vinegar

juice of ½ lemon

1 tablespoon sesame oil

1 tablespoon tamari

½ teaspoon chili powder

4 ounces spinach

Place the cauliflower steaks in a single layer on a large baking sheet. Whisk all the remaining cauliflower ingredients together in a bowl with 2 tablespoons water to make a dressing. Pour this over the cauliflower and turn to make sure each steak is evenly coated. Let marinate for at least 1 hour.

Preheat the oven to 350°F. Roast for about 40 minutes, or until tender, turning every so often.

Meanwhile, make the quinoa. Place the quinoa in a saucepan with 2 cups water and a little salt. Cover, bring to a boil, then reduce the heat and simmer for 12–15 minutes, until tender.

Mix the cilantro and chile. Scoop the avocado into a bowl and mash. Mix in the cilantro and chile, the olive oil, vinegar, lemon juice, sesame oil and tamari. Season well and stir in the chili powder.

Once the quinoa is cooked, stir in the spinach so that it wilts a little, then stir in the avocado mixture.

Place each cauliflower steak on a bed of quinoa and add a big dollop of Sun-Dried Tomato & Butter Bean Hummus.

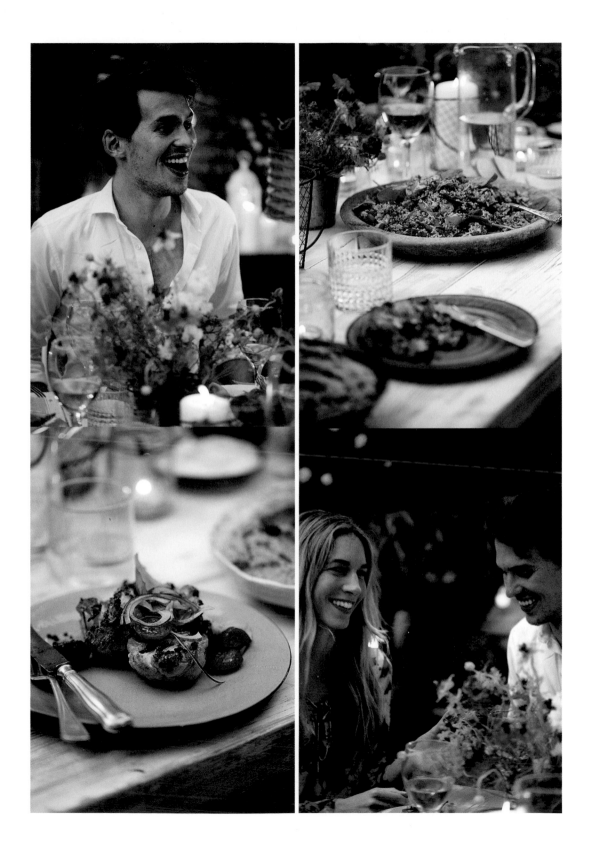

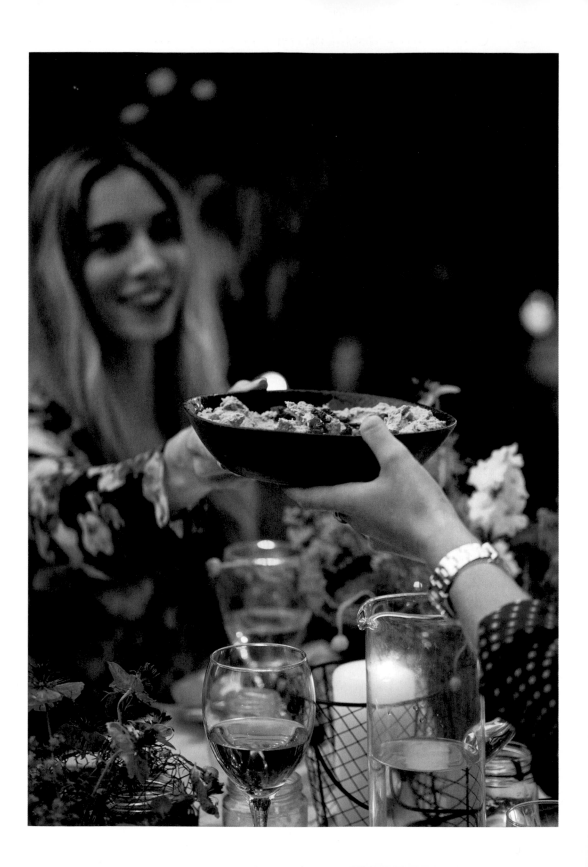

SUN-DRIED TOMATO & BUTTER BEAN HUMMUS

As many of you might know by now, I am a hummus addict: it's my all-time favorite food and something I eat pretty much every day. As a result I'm always looking for new and improved ways to make it, and this version is incredible. It's a great dish for sharing with friends, too. I normally have a bowl ready and waiting for them when they arrive for dinner. The butter beans make the hummus especially creamy, while the sun-dried tomatoes add a wonderfully rich flavor. This tastes absolutely delicious with the Marinated Cauliflower Steaks (page 134) as it really complements the mix of spices in that dish, but it also tastes amazing with simple crackers and crudités as a snack. I normally make extra, so I can keep a bowl in the fridge and enjoy it all week.

Makes a very large bowlful

NUT-FREE

two 15-ounce cans butter beans (or lima
    beans), drained and rinsed
one 10-ounce jar oil-packed sun-dried
    tomatoes, drained (6 ounces drained weight)
2 tablespoons tahini
juice of 2 lemons
2 teaspoons ground cumin
2 tablespoons olive oil
½ tablespoon apple cider vinegar
salt and pepper

Simply place all the ingredients in a food processer with 3½ tablespoons water and blend until smooth and creamy. Season to taste

Store any leftovers in an airtight jar in the fridge; they will keep well for 5–7 days.

SUPER SPEEDY
10 minutes

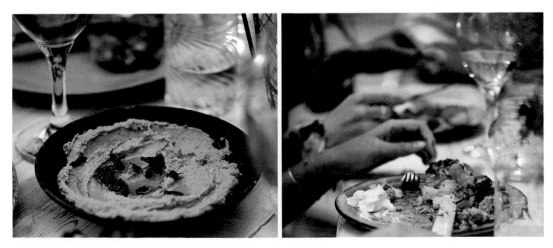

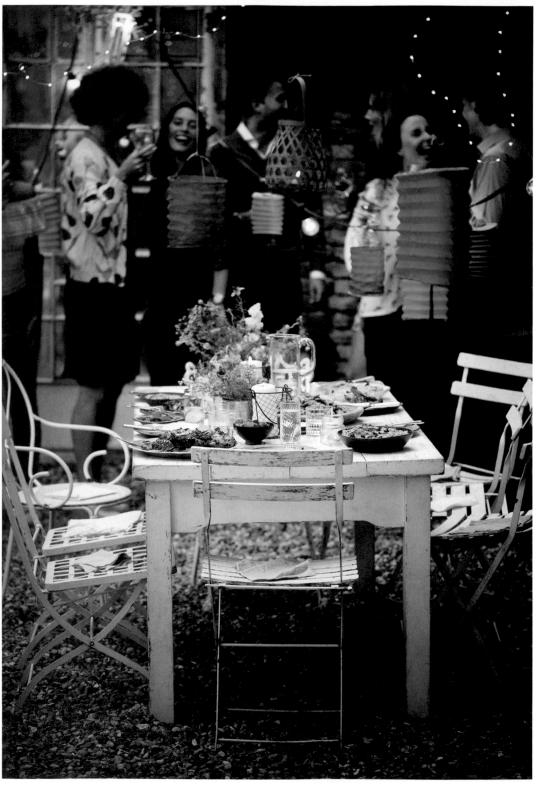

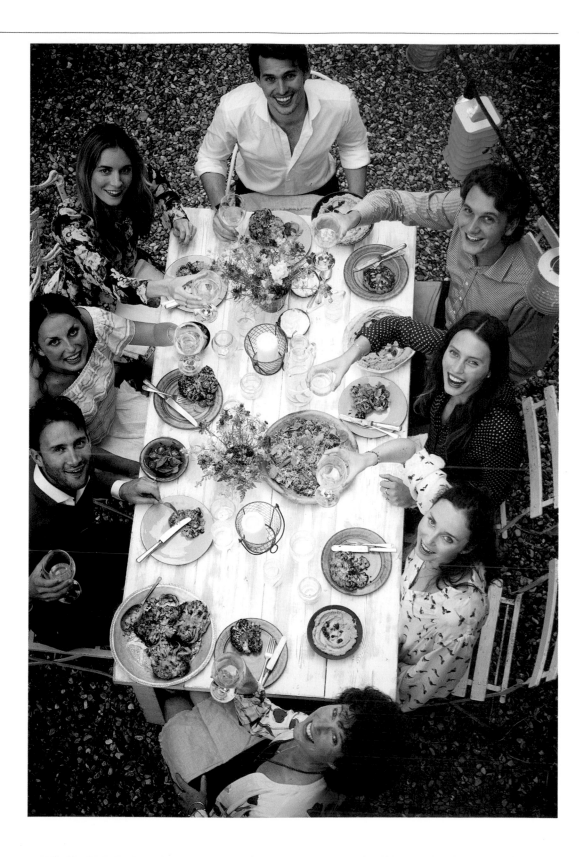

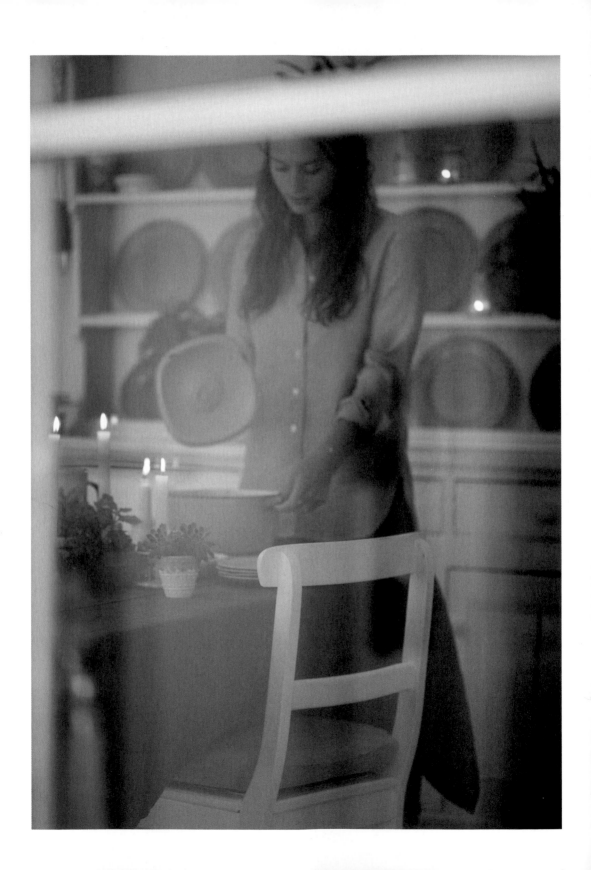

THREE-BEAN STEW

*As soon as autumn arrives and the weather cools down, I start making this all the time.
It's a warming, hearty dish that tastes lovely served on a bed of hot brown rice or quinoa
with a big dollop of Mango Salsa on top (page 143). I love the mix of black, butter and
cannellini beans; they create such a fantastic mix of textures that satisfies me every time.
This is very freezable, so you can make a larger quantity and keep the rest to enjoy as
a healthy ready meal for when you're busy. I never used to eat much onion, as it didn't
agree with me, but I've been slowly reintroducing it to my diet . . . which is why you're
now seeing more of it, too. If you're not an onion person, feel free to leave it out.*

Serves 6

NUT-FREE
olive oil
2 celery stalks, finely chopped
1 medium onion (optional), finely chopped
salt and pepper
4 garlic cloves, finely chopped
2 fresh red chiles, seeded and finely
   chopped
one 14.5-ounce can diced tomatoes
4 tablespoons tomato paste
2 red bell peppers, finely chopped
one 15-ounce can each of butter beans
   (lima beans), black beans and cannellini
   beans, drained and rinsed
large handful of cilantro

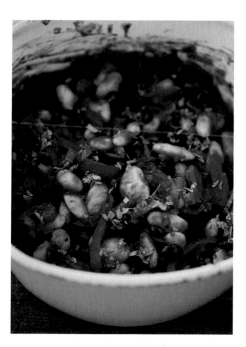

Heat a large glug of oil in a large saucepan
over medium heat. Add the celery and onion
(if using) with lots of salt and pepper and stir
until the celery is turning translucent. Add
the garlic and chiles and cook for a minute,
stirring so that nothing catches.

Add the canned tomatoes, tomato paste, bell
peppers and 1½ cups water and let it bubble
for about 30 minutes, stirring to break down
the tomatoes now and then, until the sauce is
starting to reduce and the peppers are soft.

Once you're ready to eat, add the beans.
They'll need about 10 minutes. When they've
had that, remove from the heat and let cool
slightly.

Serve in bowls with some Mango Salsa (page
143) mixed into each serving, topped with a
sprinkling of cilantro.

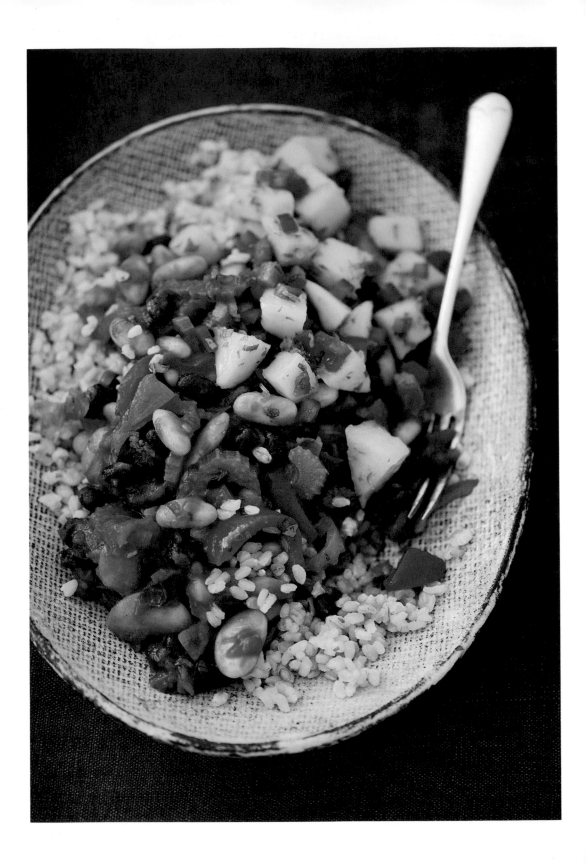

MANGO SALSA

It may sound weird to add a mango salsa to a bean stew, but trust me, it tastes incredible. It's a lovely twist to the recipe that gives a zing to each bite. It sweetens it and freshens it up, while also adding great color, which makes the dish look much more beautiful, so your friends and family will want to devour the whole thing! You can also use this to add zip to Smoky Baked Tortilla Chips or as a summery filling for Quesadillas (pages 199 and 110). If you like onion, try a little very finely chopped sweet red onion mixed in, too, to add a little bite.

Serves 6

NUT-FREE

3 mangoes

1 red bell pepper

1 jalapeño or other chile, seeded and finely chopped

juice of 2 limes

1 teaspoon apple cider vinegar

3 tablespoons olive oil

salt

small handful of cilantro leaves, finely chopped

Peel and chop the mangoes into bite-size pieces. Chop the bell pepper into small pieces (you want these to be smaller than the mango pieces).

Mix the mangoes, bell pepper, jalapeño, lime juice, vinegar, olive oil and salt to taste in a bowl. Stir well so everything is coated in oil and lime juice.

Sprinkle the cilantro on top.

SUPER SPEEDY

10 minutes

CHICKPEA CHILI IN BAKED SWEET POTATOES

This is one of my go-to easy meals. It is easy to throw together and you just need a couple of fresh ingredients to make it; everything else is a pantry essential, so you save money and put what you already have to good use. I promise it's still bursting with flavor though, thanks to the blend of spices, miso, garlic and chiles. I love cooking big batches of this to serve with a big pile of Spiced Roast Cauliflower on the side (page 149); it's such a warming, comforting meal and great to serve to a bunch of hungry friends. I freeze any chili leftovers to make sure I always have some healthy instant meals on hand. If you want to eat more quickly, use quinoa instead of baked sweet potatoes, as quinoa only takes about fifteen minutes to cook.

Serves 4

FOR THE POTATOES

4 medium sweet potatoes, scrubbed well

olive oil

flaky sea salt

FOR THE CHILI

olive oil

2 fresh red chiles, finely chopped

2 celery stalks, finely chopped

4 garlic cloves, crushed

1 teaspoon miso paste

2 teaspoons mustard seeds

2 teaspoons paprika

2 teaspoons ground cumin

½ teaspoon chili powder

salt and pepper

2 cups cherry tomatoes, quartered

one 14.5-ounce can diced tomatoes

3 tablespoons tomato paste

two 15-ounce cans chickpeas,
    drained and rinsed

2 tablespoons apple cider vinegar

7 ounces spinach

coconut yogurt, to serve

Preheat the oven to 425°F. Line a baking sheet with parchment paper.

Pierce the sweet potatoes all over, making small cuts to make sure the air can escape as they bake. Pour a little olive oil into your hands and rub the sweet potatoes all over so they have a thin coating. Place them on the baking sheet and sprinkle them evenly on all sides with sea salt.

Pop them in the oven and bake for 1 hour, or until tender inside.

Meanwhile, make the chili. Heat a generous glug of olive oil, the chiles and celery in a large frying pan over medium-high heat. Add the garlic, miso, mustard seeds, paprika, cumin, salt and pepper. Let this cook for about 5 minutes, or until the celery has softened.

Add the cherry tomatoes, canned tomatoes and tomato paste, then carefully stir in the chickpeas and vinegar.

Let everything cook for about 30 minutes. When you're ready to eat, stir in the spinach to wilt. Check the seasoning again. Split the baked sweet potatoes and serve with the chili and a dollop of yogurt.

MIX IT UP
Try baked sweet potatoes filled with Maple & Rosemary Butter Beans (page 51).

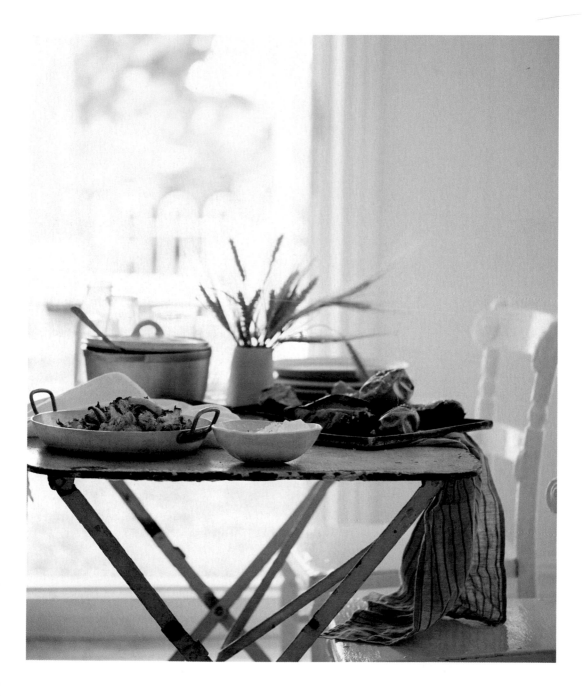

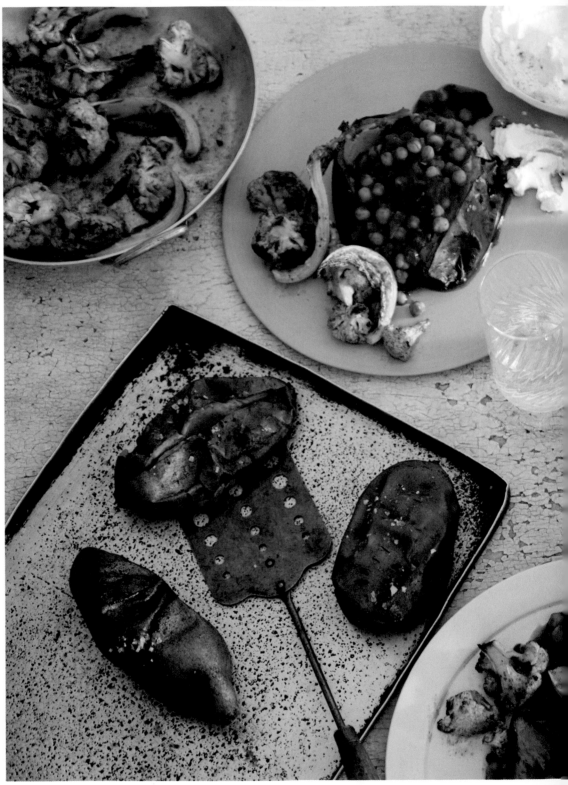

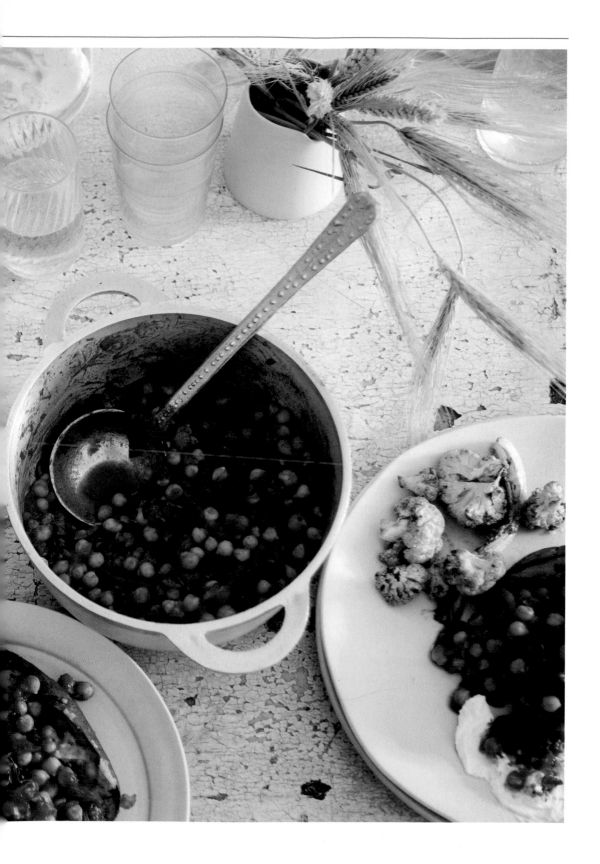

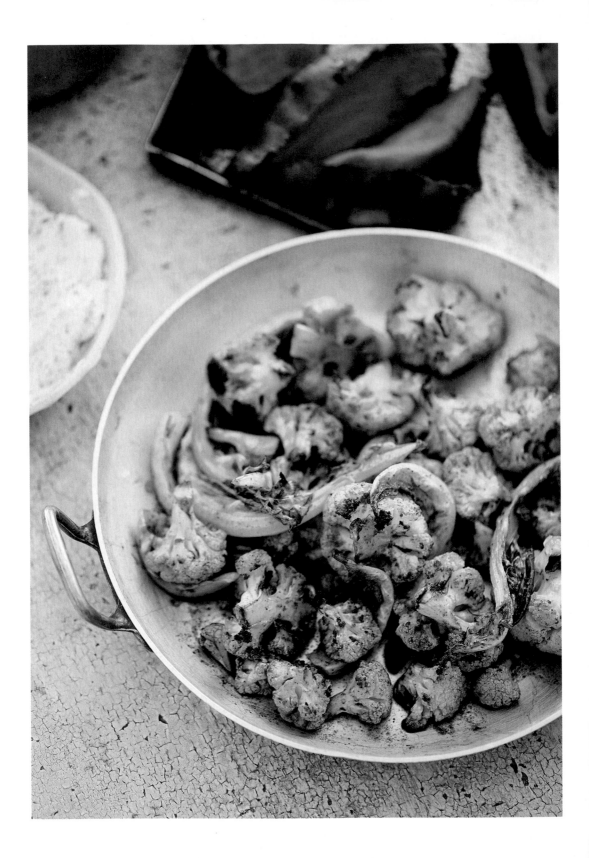

SPICED ROAST CAULIFLOWER

Cauliflower is one of the best vegetables because it's so versatile. It's particularly delicious when it's roasted with lots of warming spices until it turns golden brown and slightly crispy; like this, it's almost unbeatable. The spices do wonders here to make sure that every bite is bursting with flavor, plus they really complement the spices used in the Chickpea Chili (page 144), which is why the dishes go so well together.

Serves 4 as a side dish

NUT-FREE

3 tablespoons olive oil

1 teaspoon ground turmeric

½ teaspoon cayenne pepper

½ teaspoon ground cumin

salt and lots of pepper

1 head cauliflower, broken into florets

Preheat the oven to 425°F.

In a large bowl, whisk together the oil and the spices. Toss in the cauliflower florets. Use spoons to toss if you'd prefer not to get turmeric all over your fingers! (It can stain them yellow.) The cauliflower florets should be coated all over in the spiced oil.

Pour the spicy cauliflower out onto a baking sheet and roast for 35–40 minutes, until the pieces are golden brown.

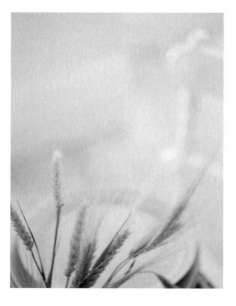

MY FAVORITE CURRIED VEGGIES

The best meal for a cozy night snuggled on the sofa. Each mouthful is immensely flavorful, as the carrots, peppers, cauliflower, peas and spinach are cooked in an amazing blend of coconut milk and spices. I love serving this in a big bowl with a bed of hot brown rice under the curry and a good dollop of my Lime & Chile Pickle on the side (page 153). This tastes even better the next day, if you don't finish it all in one sitting.

Serves 3–4 generously

1 medium head cauliflower, broken into similar-size florets

4 tablespoons olive oil

salt and pepper

4 carrots, peeled and sliced on the diagonal into 1-inch chunks

2 red bell peppers, cut into 1-inch chunks

2 tablespoons cumin seeds

5 garlic cloves, finely grated

2 inches fresh ginger, finely grated

1 tablespoon ground coriander

1 tablespoon curry powder

2 teaspoons ground cumin

½ teaspoon ground turmeric

5 whole cloves

3 tablespoons tomato paste

one 14.5-ounce can diced tomatoes

one 14-ounce can coconut milk

2 fresh green finger chiles

juice of ½ lemon, or to taste

7 ounces fresh baby spinach

¾ cup frozen peas

large handful of cilantro leaves, chopped, to serve

Preheat the oven to 410°F. Place the cauliflower on a baking sheet, drizzle with 1 tablespoon of the oil, season with salt and pepper and give them a mix to evenly coat. Place the carrots and bell peppers on a second baking sheet, drizzle with 1 tablespoon of the oil, season with salt and pepper and the cumin seeds and mix it all with your hands. Roast both sheets for 45 minutes. Check every 10 minutes or so, and give them a shake; you want the carrots and peppers to shrivel and sweeten, and the cauliflower to blacken a little and take on a gorgeous roasted flavor.

Meanwhile, in a high-sided pot, gently heat the remaining 2 tablespoons olive oil over medium heat. Add the garlic and ginger with a pinch of salt and stir so it cooks a little but doesn't color. Once they give off a lovely scent, add the dry spices and stir, still making sure not to burn anything. Stir in the tomato paste. Add the canned tomatoes and coconut milk. Bring to a boil and simmer gently. Add the green chiles. If you're like me and enjoy spicy food, slice them open and leave the seeds in; however, for a milder curry, throw them in whole. The longer you leave it simmering, the more delicious it will taste, but I cook it for at least 30 minutes.

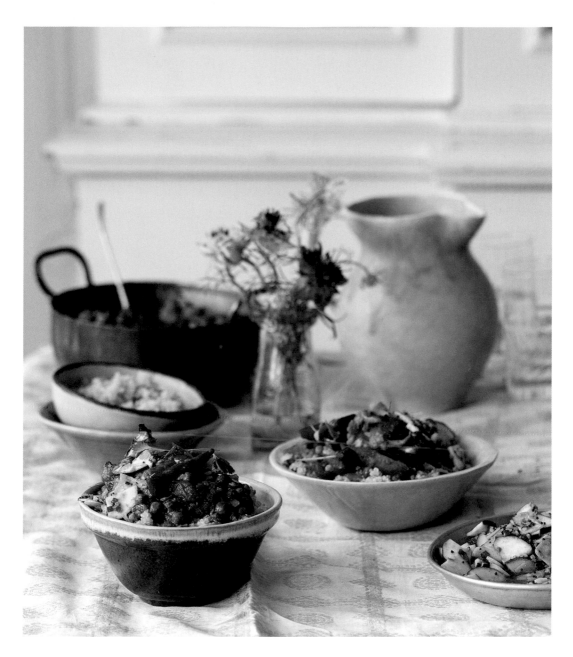

When there are just 5 minutes before you want to eat, taste the curry and add lemon juice to heighten the flavors. Stir in the spinach and peas. They should take about 2 minutes to wilt and heat through. Finally, stir in the roasted vegetables, being careful not to break the cauliflower florets apart too much. Serve with brown rice or quinoa, sprinkling with lots of cilantro before eating.

CLEVER COOKING
I don't bother to peel ginger, just grate it straight into the pan.

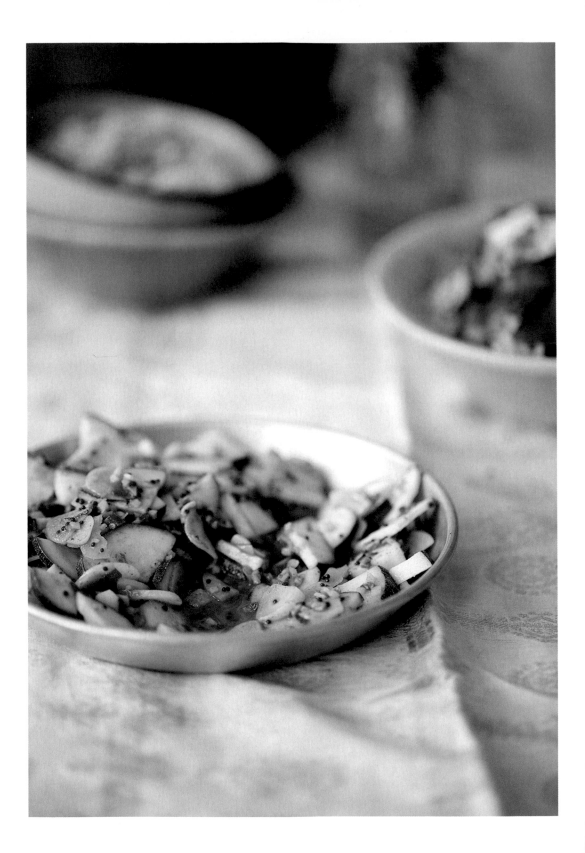

LIME & CHILE PICKLE

This is a great addition to My Favorite Curried Veggies (page 150); it really brings out so much of the flavor and heightens all the amazing essences of the meal. The mix of mustard and fenugreek seeds with the other spices is just incredible, especially with the zesty lime and apple cider vinegar. I'm sure you'll love the taste of this. You can add a dollop to any meal, not only a curry, to add an extra punch to a simple dish.

Serves 3–4

NUT-FREE

1 teaspoon mustard seeds
½ teaspoon fenugreek seeds
8 garlic cloves, thinly sliced
knob of fresh ginger, peeled and finely chopped
1–2 fresh red chiles (depending on how spicy you like it), chopped
2 tablespoons sesame oil
1 teaspoon ground turmeric
1 teaspoon chili powder
1 teaspoon ground coriander
juice of 3 limes
2 tablespoons apple cider vinegar
1 zucchini, quartered lengthwise and thinly sliced crosswise

Place a frying pan over medium heat and dry-fry the mustard seeds and fenugreek seeds for about 2 minutes, or until fragrant. Set aside in a bowl.

Add the garlic, ginger and chiles to the frying pan with the sesame oil. Cook, stirring continuously, for about 5 minutes, or until the garlic and ginger are cooked through and just starting to brown.

Add the mustard seeds, fenugreek seeds, ground spices, lime juice and vinegar and cook for another minute.

Add the zucchini (you can add 1 tablespoon of water if things are starting to stick), and cook for 6–8 minutes, until cooked through.

Remove from the heat and allow to cool before serving.

CLEVER COOKING

If by any chance you have made the pickle too spicy, then add a cooling dollop of coconut yogurt. It tastes delicious and is far more effective than water for removing chile burn.

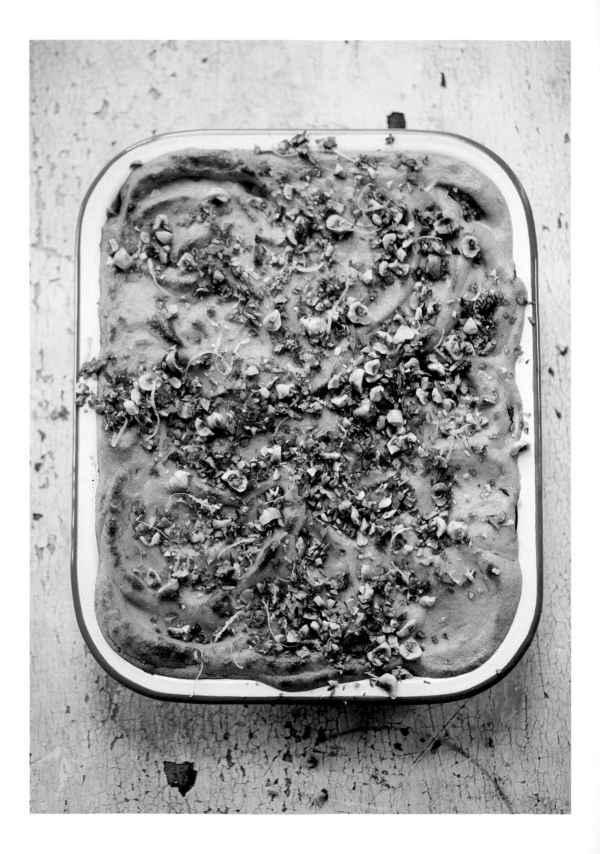

TOMATO & EGGPLANT BAKE

This is one of my favorite recipes in the book; it's really very special and I'd recommend you all trying it as soon as you can! The "cheesy" layer, which was inspired by the amazing Serena in my office, is the best part. It makes each bite so creamy and rich, warming and comforting . . . perfect for a cold evening with friends. I find this filling enough on its own, so I normally just make a side of Spinach with Mustard Seeds (page 156) to sit alongside it, but it's great with some hot quinoa, too.

Serves 6–8

2 large eggplants

salt and pepper

2 zucchini

3 tablespoons olive oil, plus more to brush

1 fennel bulb, finely chopped

3 red bell peppers, roughly chopped

6 garlic cloves, crushed

4 teaspoons smoked paprika

three 14.5-ounce cans diced tomatoes

2 tablespoons tomato paste

one 10-ounce jar oil-packed sun-dried tomatoes (6 ounces drained weight), drained and chopped

a few sprigs of fresh thyme

1 teaspoon chili flakes

scant ¾ cup hazelnuts

finely grated zest of 1 unwaxed lemon

1 ounce flat-leaf parsley, leaves picked and finely chopped

FOR THE CHEESY SAUCE

7 ounces butternut squash (about one-third of a squash), peeled and roughly chopped

generous 1 cup cashews, soaked in water for at least 4 hours, then drained

2 tablespoons nutritional yeast

1 tablespoon tamari

½ teaspoon cayenne pepper (optional)

juice of 1 lemon

Preheat the oven to 350°F.

Slice the eggplants lengthwise into slices roughly ¼ inch thick, place on 2 baking sheets in a single layer, sprinkle liberally with salt and set aside to let water draw out. Slice the zucchini lengthwise into ¼-inch slices too.

Place a grill pan over high heat. Brush it with olive oil and start grilling the zucchini slices. Lay them on gently and leave them until you can see the grill lines coming through the top side. Set aside. Keep going until all the zucchini slices are done.

Heat the 3 tablespoons of olive oil in a large nonstick frying pan over medium heat. Add the fennel, season with salt and pepper and cook for 3 minutes. Add the peppers and garlic and cook for 3 minutes. Add the paprika, stirring to coat. Now tip in the canned tomatoes, tomato paste, sun-dried tomatoes, thyme and chili flakes. Let the tomato sauce simmer and reduce for at least 20 minutes.

Meanwhile, you can get on with the eggplants. Using paper towels, brush off the salt and water from the eggplant slices, and start grilling on the hot grill pan (make sure you have your exhaust fan on! It gets smoky

>>

but the flavor makes it worthwhile). Grill for about 1 minute each side, and set aside. Once the eggplants are all done, the tomato sauce should have reduced by one-third, look glossy and coat the back of a spoon nicely. If this is so, you can start assembling the bake. Check the sauce for seasoning and add more salt and pepper if needed.

Place the hazelnuts on a baking sheet and bake for 7–10 minutes, until they turn golden. Set aside to cool.

Take a lasagne dish and put a layer of eggplant on the bottom, followed by a layer of tomato sauce, then a layer of zucchini. Keep layering until everything is used up, finishing with a layer of the tomato sauce.

Cover with foil and bake on the middle rack of the oven for 30 minutes.

Meanwhile, make the cheesy sauce. Steam the squash for 15 minutes. Add to a high-powered blender with the remaining sauce ingredients and blend until totally smooth, seasoning very well.

Remove the foil from the bake, pour over the sauce and return to the oven for another 10 minutes.

Meanwhile, chop the hazelnuts and mix in a bowl with the lemon zest and parsley.

Remove the bake from the oven, sprinkle half of the herby nut mixture over the top and take to the table to serve. Put the rest of the hazelnut mixture in a bowl on the table so people can add extra to their plate should they want it.

CLEVER COOK

Keep lemons after you have zested them to slice and use in drinks, such as in a big pitcher of water for the table.

SPINACH WITH MUSTARD SEEDS

I love serving a big bowl of this hot, wilted spinach as a side in the winter. Sautéing the spinach with mustard seeds, garlic, lemon and ginger gives it so much flavor, but the quantities of each ingredient aren't huge so the taste isn't overpowering, allowing the dish to always complement your main. I think it's the perfect addition to my favorite Tomato & Eggplant Bake (page 155), plus it adds another portion of veg to the meal, which means you can get the goodness from six different veggies!

Serves 6

NUT-FREE

20 ounces "adult" (not baby leaf) spinach

3 tablespoons olive oil

1 tablespoon mustard seeds

3 garlic cloves, crushed

2½ inches fresh ginger, finely grated

juice of 1½ lemons

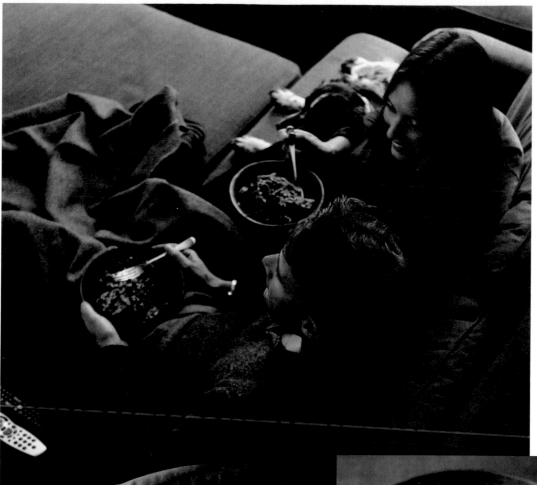

First rinse the spinach, then roughly chop it.

Heat the oil in a large frying pan. Once it's hot, add the mustard seeds and cook them until they start to pop, then add the garlic and ginger and stir for about 1 minute, making sure the garlic doesn't color.

Throw in the spinach and squeeze in the lemon juice, cook until the spinach is wilted, then enjoy straightaway.

SUPER SPEEDY
10 minutes

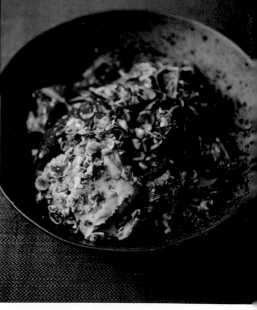

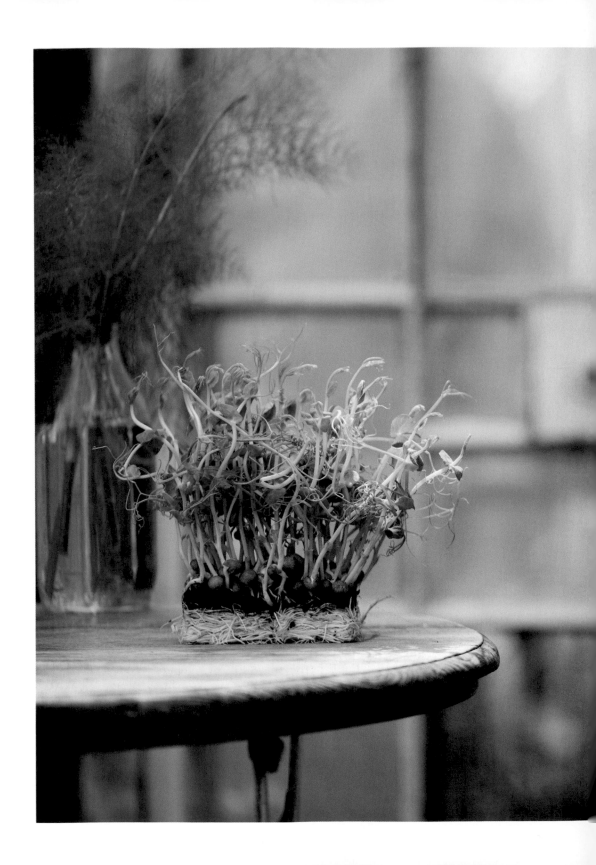

SIDES

VIBRANT BOWLS OF GOODNESS TO ADD TO ANY MEAL

WHOLE ROASTED CUMIN & DATE CARROTS

I had the most amazing whole roasted carrots with dates in a restaurant in LA a few years ago, and I loved them so much that I had to recreate them the next day and have made them many times since. I add a little maple syrup to the carrots as they roast to enhance their sweetness, plus some paprika and cumin to intensify the flavors. These taste amazing with everything, but they're particularly good alongside the Miso & Sesame Glazed Eggplants (page 173). If you can get carrots in different colors, they look great.

Serves 4 as a side dish

NUT-FREE

16 small carrots (about 1½ pounds), I use carrots with the tops still on because they look nice, peeled or well scrubbed

olive oil

1 tablespoon maple syrup

1 teaspoon ground cumin

1 teaspoon cumin seeds

1 teaspoon paprika

salt

4 medjool dates, pitted and roughly chopped

Preheat the oven to 425°F.

Place the carrots on a rimmed baking sheet, drizzle with a generous amount of olive oil, the maple syrup, both types of cumin, the paprika and salt. Toss the carrots to make sure they're evenly coated.

Roast for about 30 minutes, giving the carrots a shake halfway through.

Take the sheet out of the oven, add the dates and mix gently, then return to the oven for a final 10 minutes, after which the carrots should be golden, sweet and delicious . . . and a tad wrinkly.

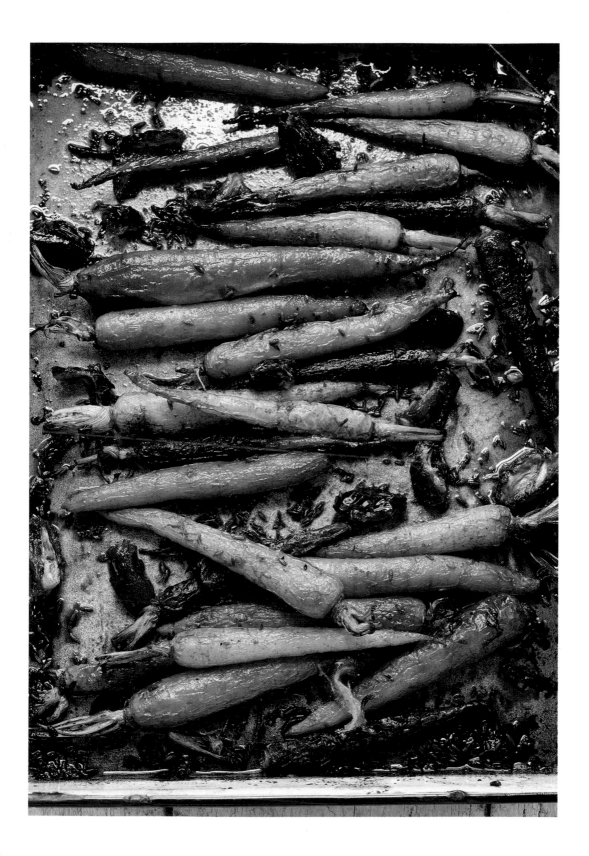

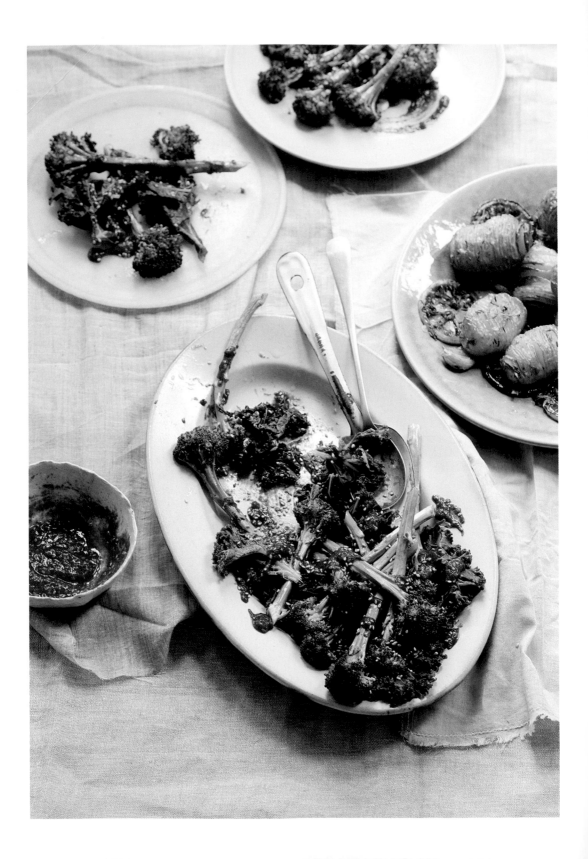

HARISSA & SESAME GREENS

This is my absolute best way to eat greens; the mix of sesame and harissa just makes them so delicious. Each bite is bursting with flavor, and the subtle spiciness does wonders for making something so simple taste really special. I eat these with so many dishes, from simple quinoa bowls to Spiced Potato Cakes with Garlicky Tomato Sauce or Herbed Nut Roast (pages 60 and 123). They also make a fantastic duo of sides with Lemony Hasselback Potatoes (page 164).

Serves 4 as a side dish

NUT-FREE

24 spears broccolini

2 tablespoons olive oil, plus more to roast

3½ cups torn-up kale, coarse ribs removed

3 tablespoons harissa

2 teaspoons sesame seeds,
    plus more to serve

juice of ½ lemon

salt

Preheat the oven to 400°F.

Place the broccolini on a baking sheet, coat with a little olive oil and toss to lightly coat. Roast for 10–15 minutes, until tender and slightly charred.

Meanwhile, steam the kale. It should take about 5 minutes. Drain well.

Mix the harissa in a bowl with the sesame seeds, lemon juice, the 2 tablespoons of olive oil and salt to taste.

Once the veg are cooked, place the kale on a plate and scatter the broccolini on top with a little more salt. Finally drizzle the harissa mixture on everything and sprinkle with a few more sesame seeds to serve.

LEMONY HASSELBACK POTATOES

I made this recipe one Christmas and it was such a hit that I wanted to share it with you all. It's a great recipe for two reasons: firstly—obviously—they taste great, as the potatoes are infused with garlic, lemon and thyme as they cook, soaking up all the flavors; but secondly they look amazing with their perfectly cut, crispy golden skin. They'll instantly impress all your guests. The good news for you is that they're actually really easy to make, as long as you have a sharp knife and a steady hand! It's simple to double (or even triple) the recipe, as we did for this photograph.

Serves 4–6 as a side dish

NUT-FREE

8 medium baking potatoes, scrubbed well, unpeeled

1 lemon

8 garlic cloves, unpeeled and squashed (bash with a rolling pin!)

leaves from 4 sprigs of fresh thyme, plus more to serve

good olive oil

flaky sea salt and pepper

Preheat the oven to 425°F.

On a cutting board, firmly hold a potato and, with a sharp knife, make cuts two-thirds of the way through it, spacing the cuts about $\frac{1}{16}$ inch apart. When you're doing this, concentrate, because you want to make sure your potato isn't cut the whole way through to the board otherwise it won't hold together. Use this time as a sort of meditation! Do this for all the spuds and then place them on a rimmed baking sheet, sliced sides up.

Halve the lemon and squeeze the juice over the potatoes. Now reshape the lemon to its original form as far as possible, slice it into rings and place on the baking sheet. Throw in the garlic and thyme. Drizzle with loads of olive oil, getting as much as you can into the cuts you've made in your spuds. Sprinkle very liberally with salt and pepper and roll everything around so that the potatoes are all nicely coated. Make sure they're all sitting sliced sides up again and put them in the oven.

After about 25 minutes, take out the lemon slices and garlic and set aside; you can eat the garlic with the potatoes later and the lemons make the dish look beautiful when presented, but if you leave them in the oven for the whole time, they will burn to a cinder.

Spoon the juices at the bottom of the baking sheet back over the potatoes and return them to the oven for another 60–65 minutes, until crispy on top and cooked through.

To serve, sprinkle with fresh thyme and return the lemon slices and garlic, if you like.

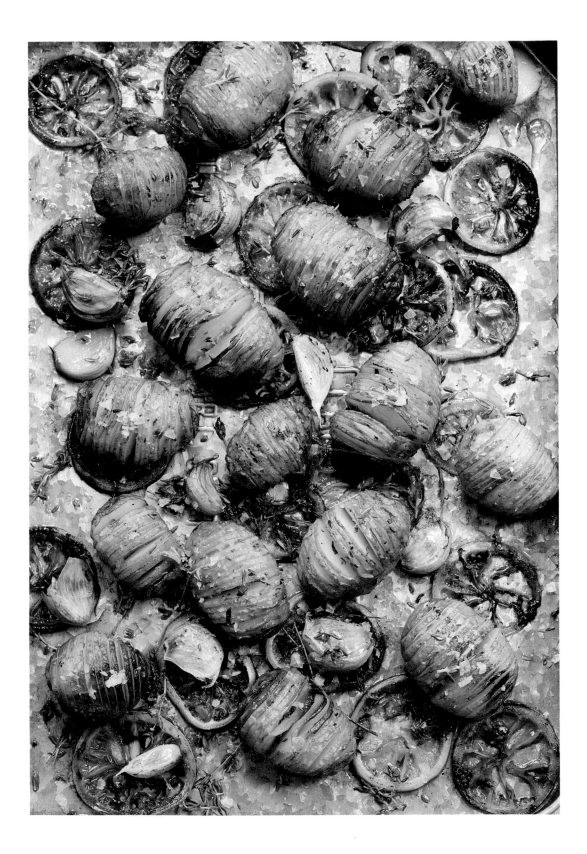

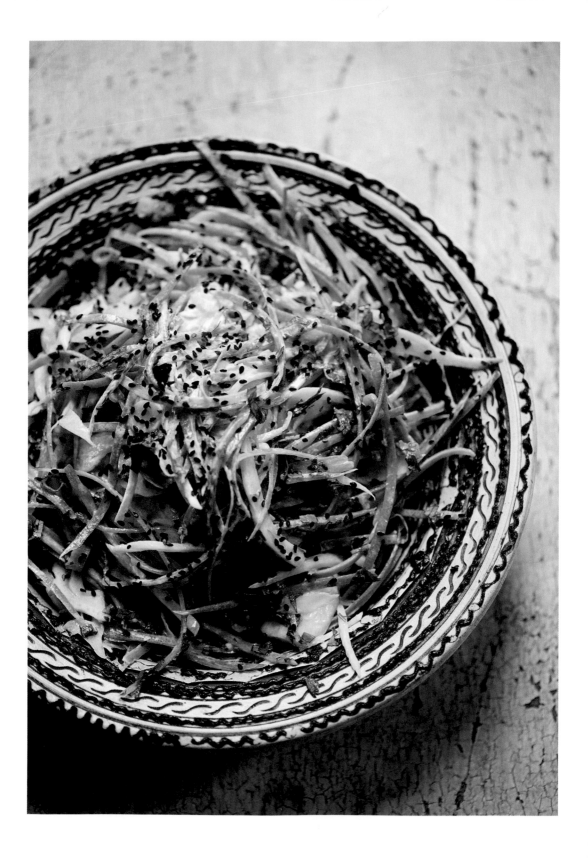

CARROT & FENNEL SLAW

This is probably the simplest, lightest recipe in this whole chapter. It's lovely and delicate, with only a handful of flavors, so that it can sit really well alongside rich dishes. I love having a side like this that I can throw together in a few minutes, to add more color and texture to the table, but without distracting from the centerpieces of a meal.

Serves 4 as a side dish

2 tablespoons olive oil
1 tablespoon sesame oil
4 tablespoons coconut yogurt
2 tablespoons apple cider vinegar
juice of ½ lemon
salt and pepper
1 small fennel bulb
2 medium carrots, peeled
4 green onions, finely chopped
2 tablespoons black sesame seeds
handful of chopped cilantro

Place the olive oil, sesame oil, yogurt, vinegar and lemon juice in a mixing bowl and whisk vigorously to make an emulsion, then season with salt and pepper.

Trim the base of the fennel bulb and, using a mandoline, slice it as thin as possible. (If you don't have a mandoline, just slice it very thinly with a knife.) Place the sliced fennel into the bowl with the dressing.

Next, slice the carrots on the mandoline, or use a shredder, so they resemble ribbons or shreds; if you don't have a mandoline, use a vegetable peeler to make ribbons. You want the carrot to retain a bit of crunch, so it's better to take the time to do this, rather than just grating it. Place in the bowl with the fennel and dressing and mix with your hands so everything is coated nicely.

Mix in the green onions. Sprinkle with the sesame seeds and chopped cilantro and serve.

SUPER SPEEDY
10 minutes

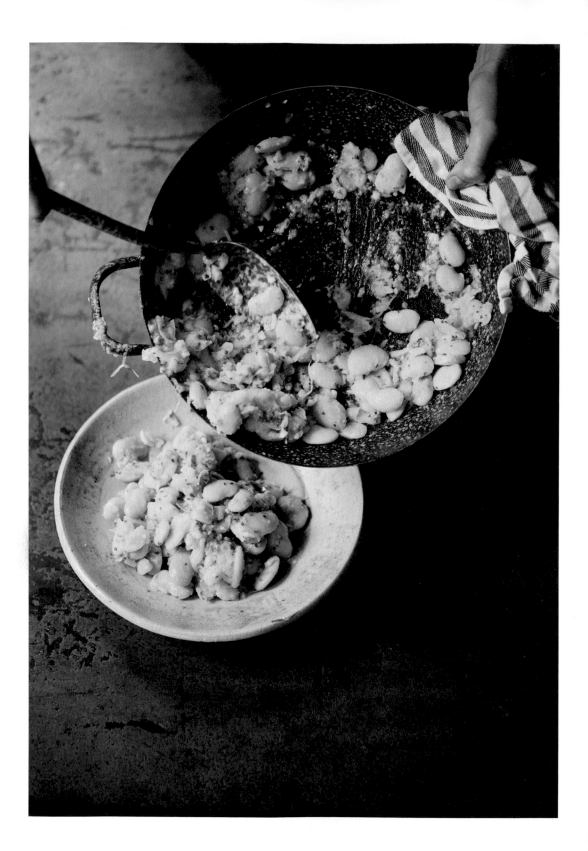

ZESTY BUTTER BEANS

This is a wonderfully simple, subtle side dish. The beans have a deliciously delicate flavor with subtle hints of rosemary, lemon and cayenne. None of the flavors is overpowering, so the beans will complement your main dish perfectly, and are especially good with my Spiced Potato Cakes with Garlicky Tomato Sauce, or Sesame, Cilantro & Roasted Fennel Rice Bowl, or with a big pile of Harissa & Sesame Greens and some Smoky Babaganoush on the side (pages 60, 104, 163 and 203).

Serves 4 as a side dish

NUT-FREE

olive oil

6 garlic cloves, crushed

6 sprigs of fresh rosemary, leaves stripped
   and roughly chopped

two 15-ounce cans butter beans (or lima
   beans), drained and rinsed

finely grated zest of 1 unwaxed lemon,
   plus the juice of 1½ lemons

½ teaspoon cayenne pepper

salt and pepper

Heat a big glug of olive oil in a saucepan over medium heat. Add the garlic and rosemary and cook for 3–5 minutes, until it's bubbling away.

Add the beans, lemon zest and juice and cayenne pepper and cook for 5–10 minutes, until the beans are soft. As you're stirring the beans, crush them slightly so you end up with a part-whole-bean-part-creamy-mash mix. Season to taste.

Drizzle with another glug of olive oil, to keep them from becoming dry, then serve.

SUPER SPEEDY

10 minutes

BLACKENED CAULIFLOWER WITH GREEN ONION PESTO

Pesto instantly adds color and flavor to anything, plus it's always so quick and easy to whizz together. As I make it so much, I love to try different variations, and this green onion version is a real winner. I can't tell you how good it tastes with the blackened cauliflower. I like to make extra pesto, so that I can keep a bowl in the fridge for a few days ready to stir into pasta or beans for a quick go-to meal.

Serves 4 as a side dish

NUT-FREE

FOR THE CAULIFLOWER

1 head cauliflower, broken into florets
olive oil
salt and pepper

FOR THE PESTO

bunch of green onions, green tops only
6 tablespoons pine nuts
½ cup fresh basil leaves
3 tablespoons nutritional yeast
1 garlic clove, crushed
juice of ½ lemon
scant ½ cup olive oil

Preheat the oven to 350°F.

Place the cauliflower florets on a rimmed baking sheet, drizzle with a little olive oil, season with salt and pepper, and pop them into the oven. Set a timer for 40 minutes, but check them every 10 minutes or so and give them a shake every now and again. You want them to blacken and char slightly on all sides.

Meanwhile, make the pesto. Bring water to a boil while you chop the green onion tops and place them in a colander. Pour boiling water over the green onion tops to wilt them.

Put the pine nuts, basil, nutritional yeast, garlic, lemon juice and wilted green onion tops into a food processor and blend to a paste. With the processor running, slowly pour in the oil. Season with salt and pepper to taste.

Once the cauliflower is cooked, serve on a platter or in a shallow dish and dollop and drizzle the pesto on top (or serve it in a bowl on the side, if you prefer). Enjoy!

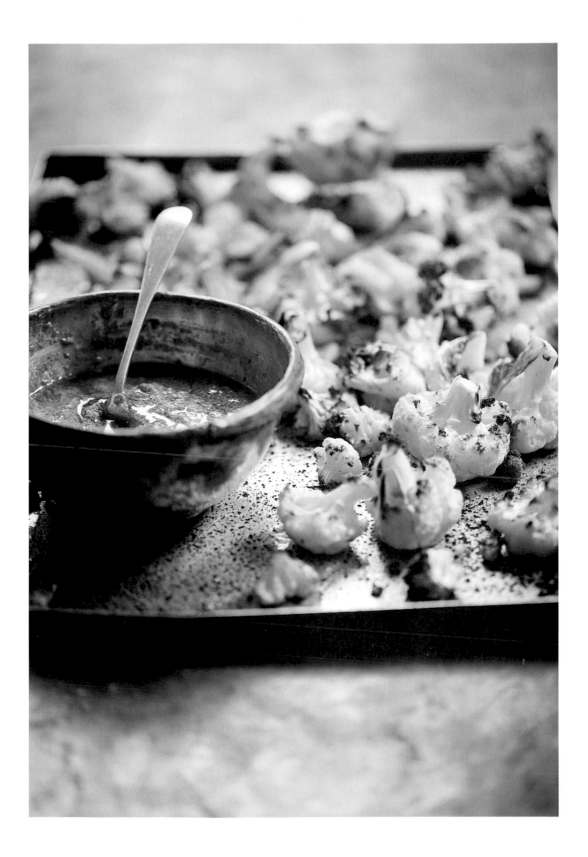

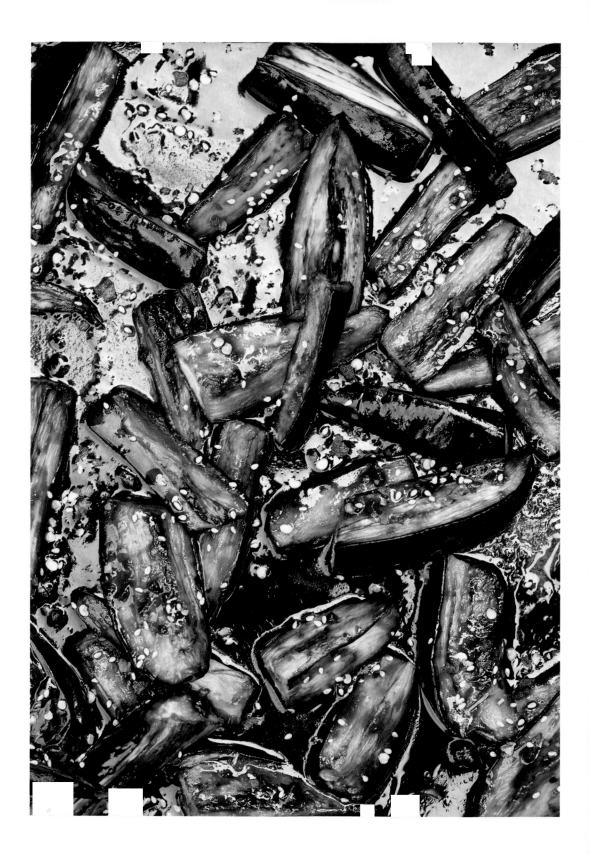

MISO & SESAME GLAZED EGGPLANT

These eggplant wedges are one of the most popular recipes I've created for this book. I've made them for so many friends and everyone goes crazy for them and asks for them again and again. They're so insanely delicious. The mix of sesame, tamari, miso, maple and lemon juice creates such rich flavors that really make each bite sing! I always make extra as everyone seems to want seconds, but also because they taste great cold, so I throw any leftovers into my lunch box the next day.

Serves 4 as a side dish

NUT-FREE

3 medium eggplants, stem ends trimmed, cut lengthwise into narrow wedges

1 tablespoon olive oil

salt

3 tablespoons sesame oil

juice of 1 lemon

1½ tablespoons tamari

1 tablespoon maple syrup

2 teaspoons brown rice miso

1 teaspoon apple cider vinegar

sesame seeds, to serve

chili flakes, to serve

Preheat the oven to 400°F.

Place the eggplant wedges on a rimmed baking sheet, drizzle with the olive oil and sprinkle with a little salt. Bake for 15–20 minutes, until soft but not completely cooked.

Meanwhile, whisk the sesame oil, lemon juice, tamari, maple syrup, miso and vinegar together in a bowl to make the glaze.

Once the wedges are soft, pour the glaze over them (while they're still on the baking sheet) and mix well. Return them to the oven to cook for another 10 minutes, then turn them over and cook for a final 5 minutes, or until they're tender and delicious and completely coated in the glaze.

Take out of the oven and sprinkle with sesame seeds and chili flakes to serve.

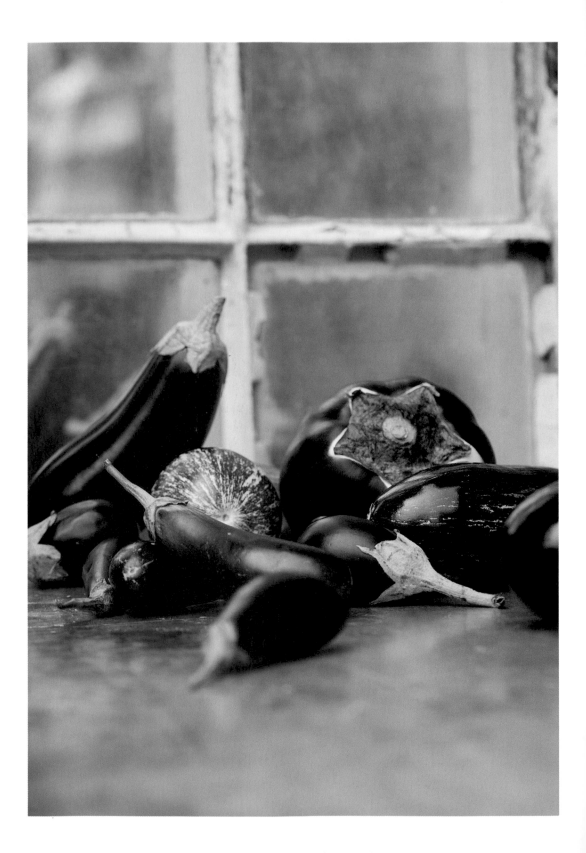

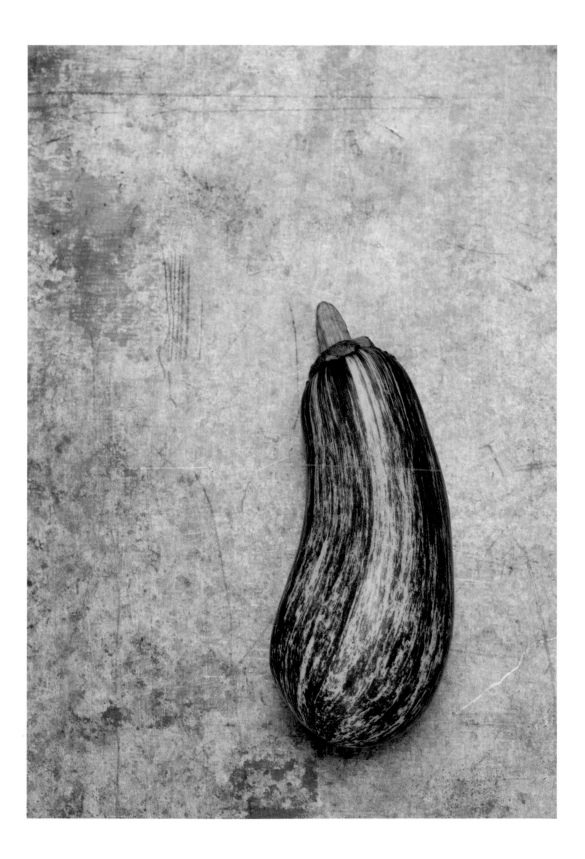

WARM MOROCCAN CAULIFLOWER "RICE" SALAD

This is a firm favorite in the Deliciously Ella office. It's inspired by the lovely Jess, in my office, and I hope you love it as much as we do. I've always been a bit skeptical about cauliflower rice, but it's growing on me and—used in this way—I think it's great. The rice is sautéed in a warming mix of spices, then tossed with roasted cashews, apricots, raisins and chickpeas, which together create something quite outstanding. I love it with Whole Roasted Cumin & Date Carrots (page 160).

Serves 4–6 as a side dish

FOR THE SALAD
¾ cup cashews
1 large head cauliflower (about 2¼ pounds)
2 tablespoons olive oil
one 15-ounce can chickpeas, drained and
    rinsed
2 teaspoons ground turmeric
2 teaspoons ground cumin
2 teaspoons cumin seeds
2 teaspoons ground coriander
1 teaspoon paprika
½ teaspoon ground cinnamon
½ teaspoon chili powder
salt and pepper
scant ½ cup raisins
1½ cups dried apricots (preferably
    unsulphured), roughly chopped
4 green onions, finely chopped
2 ounces fresh mint, leaves picked and
    chopped
2 ounces fresh flat-leaf parsley, leaves
    picked and chopped

FOR THE DRESSING
2 tablespoons tahini
1½ tablespoons olive oil
juice of ½ lemon
juice of ½ orange

Preheat the oven to 400°F. Place the cashews on a baking sheet and roast for 5–10 minutes, until they turn golden brown. Remove from the oven and let cool.

Cut the cauliflower florets from the stem and chop into 1–2-inch pieces. This makes "ricing" them much easier. Place in a food processor. Blitz until they start to resemble rice; this should take about 30 seconds.

Heat the olive oil in a large frying pan. Add the cauliflower and chickpeas, spices and salt and pepper to taste. Give it a good mix, then add the raisins, apricots and cashews. Mix in the pan for about 5 minutes until it's all warmed up. Remove the pan from the heat.

Meanwhile, whisk all the dressing ingredients in a bowl.

Check the seasoning of the cauliflower, then mix in the green onions and herbs. Drizzle with the dressing and enjoy!

MIX IT UP
I sometimes like this with a dollop of coconut yogurt and a pinch of the Moroccan spice blend *ras el hanout* on top.

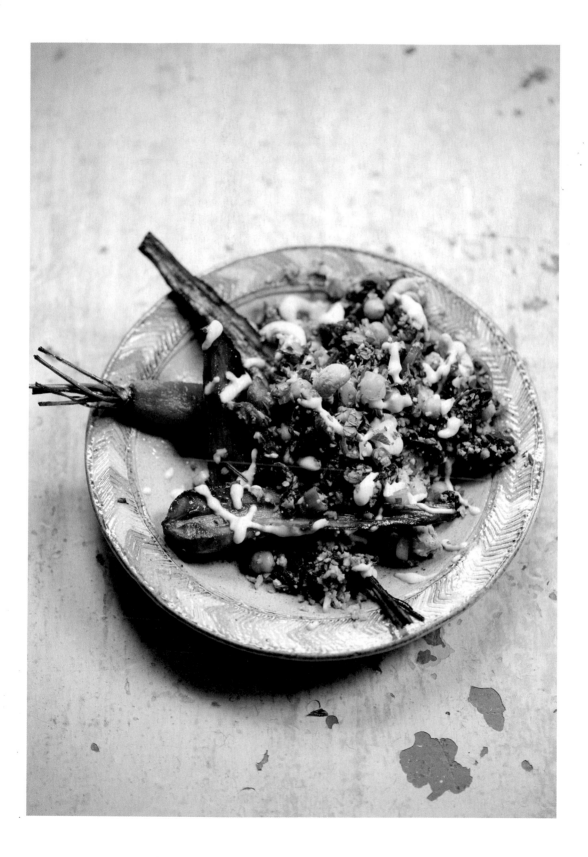

MINTY PEA PURÉE

This has been a family favorite for ages; I make it all the time when I'm at my mum's. It's another unassuming dish that doesn't require much time or effort, but the flavors are amazing. It is one of the quick fixes I reach for when I'm short on time and want to speedily make something delicious for us at home. I'll often just heat up some quinoa, roast some broccoli, sauté some beans (such as my Zesty Butter Beans, page 169), then throw it all together for a speedy supper.

Serves 4–6 as a side dish

NUT-FREE
3¾ cups frozen peas (about 18 ounces)
6 tablespoons olive oil
juice of 1½ limes, or to taste (I often
    use a little more)
small handful of fresh mint leaves
    (about 2 tablespoons), roughly chopped
salt and pepper

Place the peas in a pan of cold water. Cover and bring it to a boil, then simmer for 2 minutes. Drain, then place in a food processor with all the other ingredients.

Whizz everything together until it's fully blended. This tastes great either served warm or at room temperature.

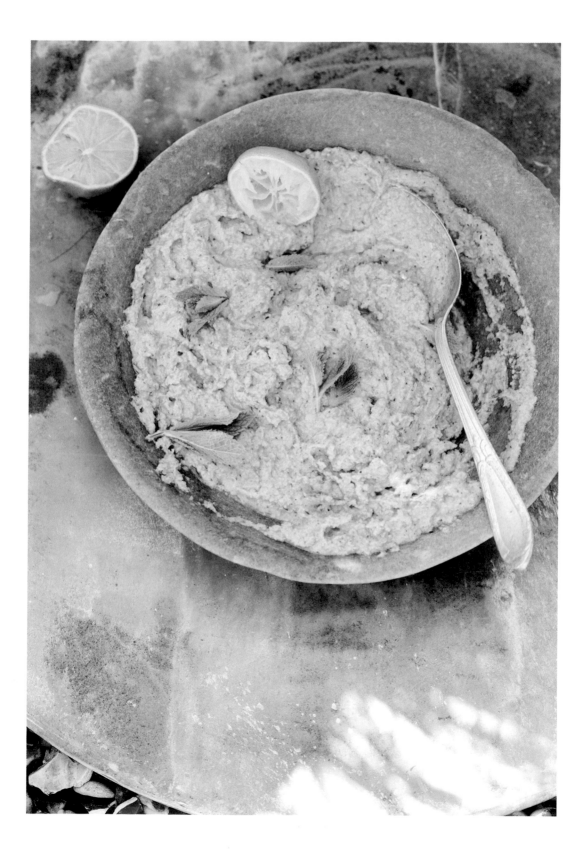

SMASHED TURMERIC & MUSTARD SEED POTATOES

This is almost my favorite dish in the chapter. Everything about these potatoes is incredibly warming and comforting; they always make me feel so grounded and happy. They are boiled and then smashed with spices, lemon juice, olive oil and lots of salt and pepper. I know lots of people stay away from potatoes, but you have to try these, they'll totally convert you into fans of the humble little spud.

Serves 4 as a side dish

NUT-FREE

2¼ pounds potatoes, peeled and
  quartered

salt and pepper

5 tablespoons olive oil

1 tablespoon mustard seeds

1 teaspoon ground turmeric

2 teaspoons ground cumin

¼ teaspoon cayenne pepper

juice of 1 lemon

Place the potatoes in a saucepan of cold water. Cover and bring to a boil, then add lots of salt. Once the water's boiling, reduce the heat and simmer for 25 minutes, or until they're soft enough to mash.

Meanwhile, heat the oil in a small saucepan over medium-high heat until it is hot. Add the mustard seeds and wait until they start popping. When this happens, add the rest of the spices, some more salt and black pepper, then finally squeeze in the lemon juice and let it bubble for a minute or so. Remove from the heat.

Once the potatoes are cooked, drain them, return them to their hot pan and roughly mash with a fork or wooden spatula. Don't let them turn into a mash, though; it's nice to keep some chunky texture here.

Stir in the spice mix and devour!

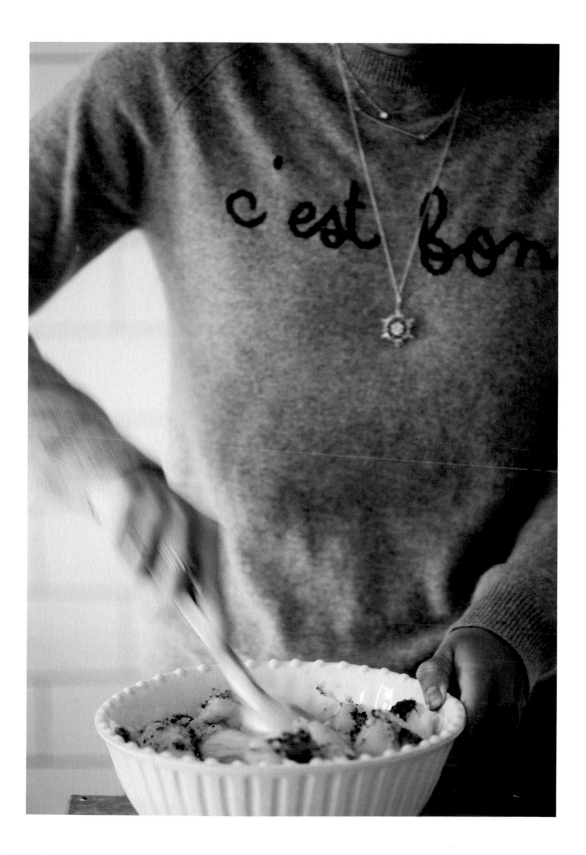

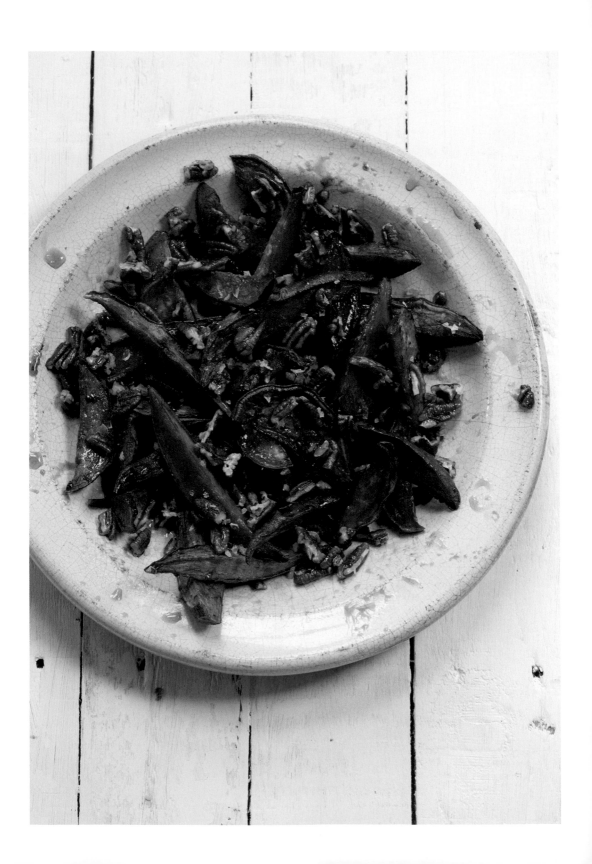

MAPLE & PECAN SWEET POTATOES

These are just a dream. They're always such a crowd-pleaser, so sweet and gooey after they've been baked with maple syrup. If you're trying to convince skeptical friends that veggies are great, then this is your dish. It's simple and totally accessible for everyone.

Serves 4 as a side dish

3 medium sweet potatoes, scrubbed well and cut into wedges
2 teaspoons ground cinnamon
2 tablespoons maple syrup
olive oil
salt and pepper
¾ cup pecans, broken into halves or quarters, depending on size

Preheat the oven to 400°F.

Put the sweet potato wedges on a baking sheet, add the cinnamon, 1 tablespoon of the maple syrup, a good glug of olive oil, and salt and pepper to taste. Mix well with your hands so all the wedges are coated.

Roast for 40–45 minutes, at which point they should be really tender. Check every so often and turn the wedges halfway through.

Meanwhile, in a small bowl, mix the pecans with the remaining 1 tablespoon maple syrup. Add the pecans to the sweet potato wedges, return to the oven and bake for another 10–15 minutes, until the nuts are golden and crunchy and the sweet potatoes soft and gooey.

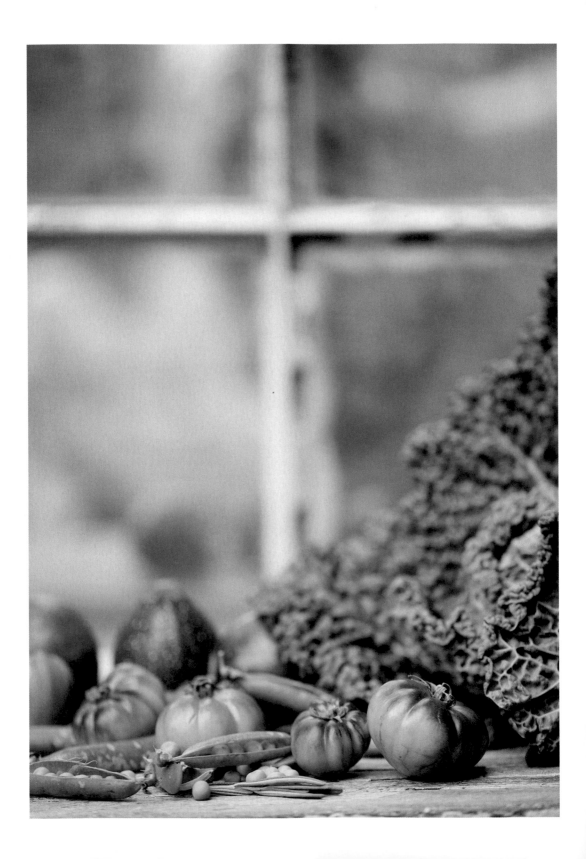

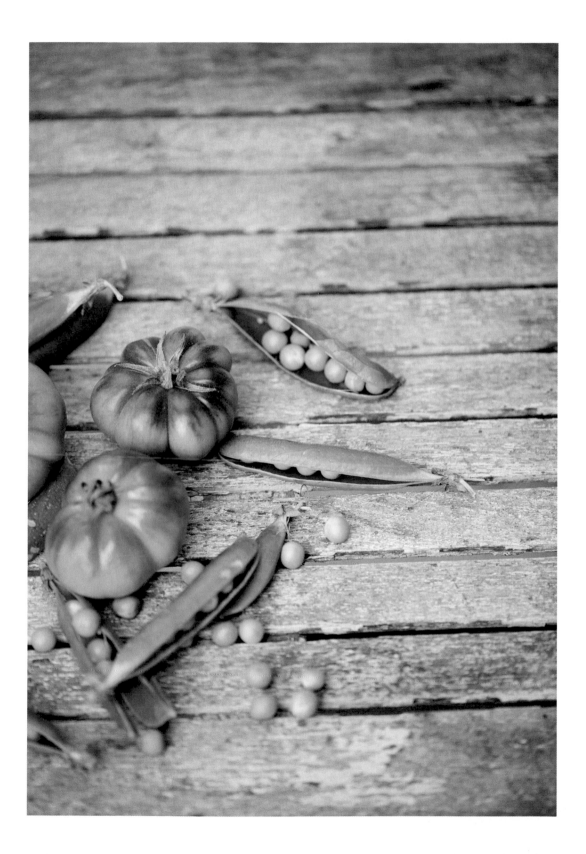

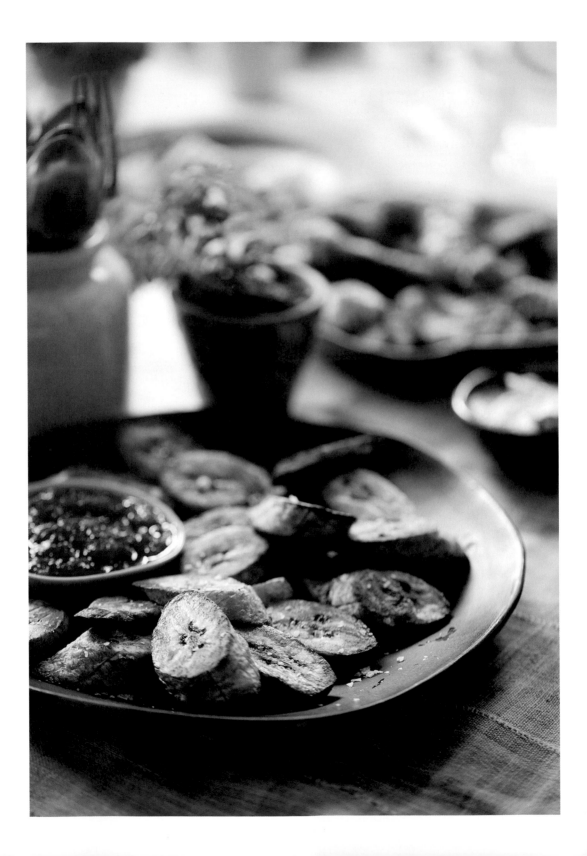

BAKED PLANTAINS WITH SWEET CHILE SAUCE

I've become totally obsessed with plantains recently, and they're now one of my absolute favorite foods. I love them simply baked until golden brown and tender with a little salt, but they are even better when drizzled with my sweet chile sauce. The two really work well together, heightening each other's natural sweetness. I've been serving these with just about everything lately, from my Sesame Slaw and Pistachio & Apricot Quinoa to My Favorite Curried Veggies (pages 99, 96 and 150).

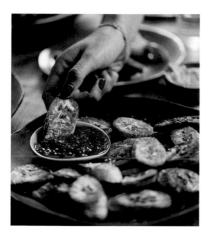

Serves 4 as a side dish

NUT-FREE

FOR THE PLANTAINS

4 plantains

olive oil

salt

FOR THE SWEET CHILE SAUCE

1 fresh red chile, seeded

1 inch fresh ginger, peeled and chopped

2 garlic cloves, halved

juice of ½ lime

½ cup honey

1 tablespoon apple cider vinegar

salt and pepper

1 teaspoon chia seeds

Preheat the oven to 400°F. Peel the plantains and cut into generous ⅓-inch-thick slices. Place in a single layer on a baking sheet. Drizzle with oil and sprinkle with salt, toss with your hands, then bake for 50 minutes to 1 hour, until golden brown, soft and tender. The longer they bake, the sweeter they get.

Meanwhile, make the sweet chile sauce. Put the chile, ginger and garlic into a food processor and blitz until finely chopped.

Squeeze the lime juice into a saucepan and add the honey, vinegar, and salt and pepper to taste. Place over medium heat, then add the chile mixture. Bring to a boil, then add the chia. Simmer for about 15 minutes, or until it thickens. Once thickened, add 2 tablespoons water, remove from the heat, scrape into a small bowl and let cool.

Either serve the plantains hot straight from the oven, or wait for them to cool and serve them at room temperature. Either way, offer lots of the sweet chile sauce on the side.

CLEVER COOKING

While plantains aren't available in every supermarket, they're generally easy to find (and often cheaper) in street markets.

SPICY BAKED AVOCADO FRIES WITH A LIME, CASHEW & CILANTRO DIP

These are an absolute revelation, my new favorite way to eat avocados and a nice change from sweet potato fries. I love the contrast of the soft, creamy chunks of avocado in the middle and the crispy, crunchy, chili coating on the outside. They're delicious dunked into this lime, cashew and cilantro dip too; or, if you want a spicy hit, try the sweet chile sauce from the plantains (page 187), which tastes amazing with these, too.

Serves 4 as a side dish

FOR THE FRIES

5 tablespoons chickpea flour

scant ¼ cup almond milk, or any other
    plant-based milk

1 tablespoon sesame oil

1 cup almond meal

¼ cup sesame seeds

2 tablespoons nutritional yeast

1 teaspoon chili flakes

¼ teaspoon chili powder

½ teaspoon paprika

¼ teaspoon cayenne pepper

½ teaspoon salt

¼ teaspoon black pepper

2 avocados, ripe but still firm

FOR THE DIP

generous ½ cup cashews, soaked for
    3 hours and drained

juice of 2½ limes

small handful of cilantro

2 tablespoons olive oil

1 tablespoon apple cider vinegar

2 sprigs of fresh mint, leaves picked

pinch of salt

Preheat the oven to 425°F. Line a baking sheet with parchment paper.

Place the chickpea flour in a bowl. Mix the almond milk and sesame oil in another bowl. Mix together the ground almonds, sesame seeds, nutritional yeast, both types of chili, paprika, cayenne, salt and black pepper in a third bowl.

Halve the avocados lengthwise, pit and peel, then slice thickly lengthwise, making about 5 slices for each avocado half.

One at a time, dip the avocado slices first in the chickpea flour, making sure it's covered. Then dip it in the milk bowl, followed by the spiced almond meal mixture. As you work, place the coated avocado slice on the prepared baking sheet.

Bake for 20 minutes, flipping halfway through.

Once the avocados are done, remove from the oven. Let cool for about 20 minutes; this helps them crisp up even more.

Meanwhile, make the dip. Combine the drained cashews, ¼ cup water and the remaining dip ingredients in a blender. Blend until really smooth.

Then dip your avocado fries into the sauce and enjoy!

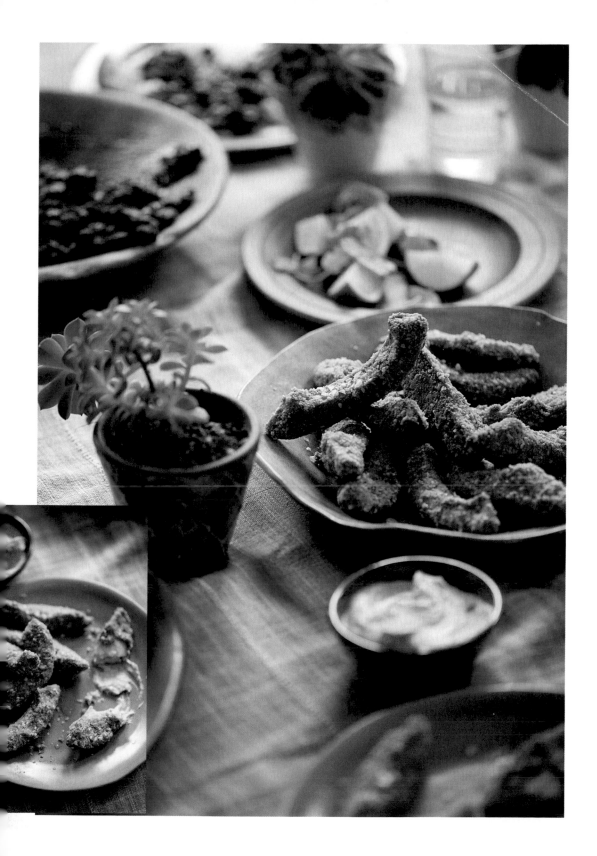

GARLICKY BLACK BEANS

These are a real staple in my diet. I find myself making the dish all the time as it's quick, and black beans are cheap and easy to get hold of. Plus this is a simple way to add a deep, rich flavor to any meal, while also making it feel heartier and more filling. I love them served with simple suppers such as brown rice and mashed avocado when I'm feeling lazy, or as a side for something a little fancier when I'm trying to impress!

Serves 4 as a side dish

NUT-FREE

5 garlic cloves, crushed

2 tablespoons olive oil

¼ teaspoon cayenne pepper

juice of 1 lemon

salt and pepper

two 15-ounce cans black beans, drained and rinsed

1 tablespoon brown rice miso paste

1 tablespoon tomato paste

Place the garlic in a saucepan with the olive oil, cayenne pepper, lemon juice and salt and black pepper to taste. Gently heat for a minute or so until it starts bubbling.

Add all the other ingredients and cook over medium heat for about 10 minutes, stirring every couple of minutes. You want the beans to be slightly softened and broken up and fully coated in the miso and tomato paste.

SUPER SPEEDY

15 minutes

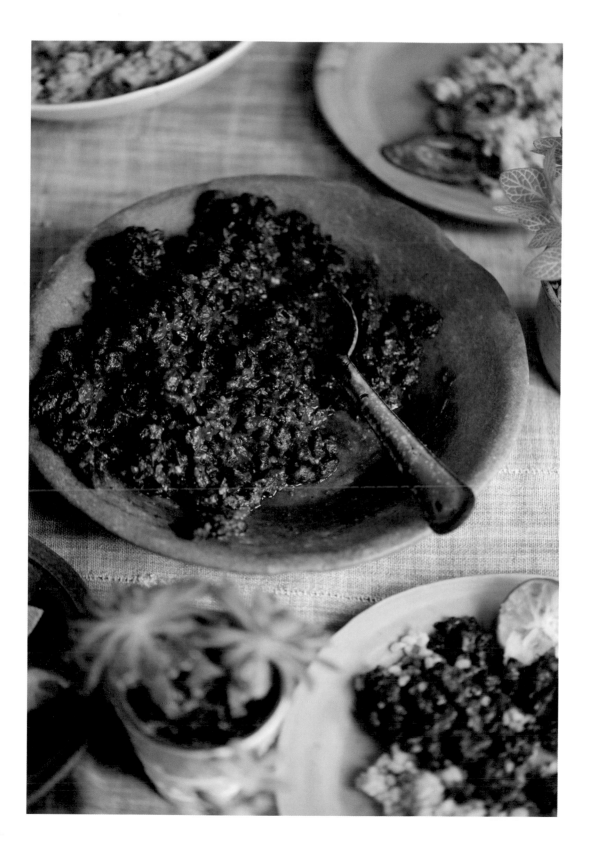

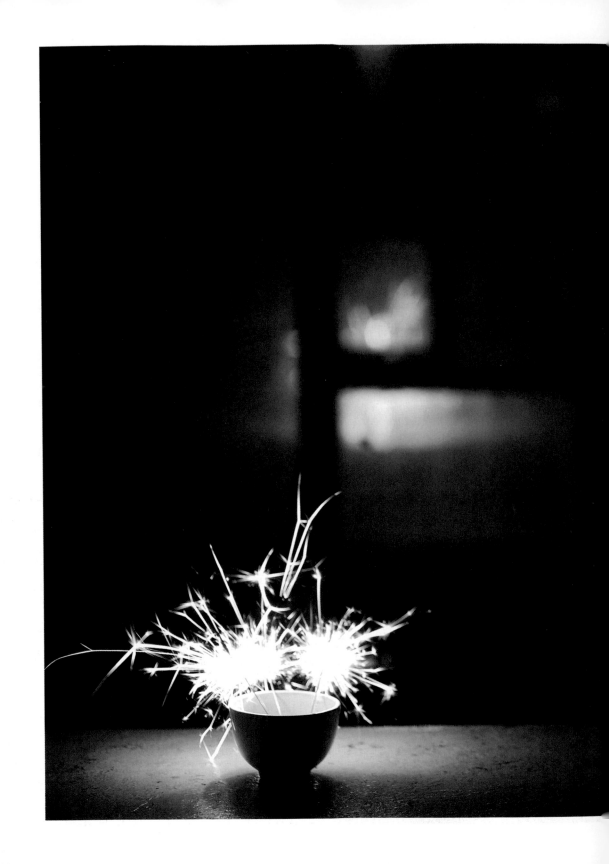

PARTIES

FUN WAYS TO SHARE YOUR FAVORITE FOODS
WITH THE PEOPLE YOU LOVE

PARTIES

Being kind to yourself with the food you eat doesn't mean that you can't have a lot of fun, and parties are absolutely not ruled out, in fact they're encouraged! You can love yourself, love your food and still have the best time with friends and family. There are so many favorites in the next few pages and it's so hard to single a few things out, but I find myself making the Beet & Sweet Potato Chips and Smoky Baked Tortilla Chips with big bowls of Smoky Babaganoush and Roast Carrot Hummus for dunking a lot. I also have the best memories of the Watermelon & Cucumber Cooler, which we served at our wedding, and of course nothing can beat a three-tiered Celebration Cake served alongside Blueberry Scones with Vanilla Coconut Cream, or a Banana & Raisin Cake!

MENUS

NIBBLES

Beet & Sweet Potato Chips
Smoky Baked Tortilla Chips
Roast Carrot Hummus
Smoky Babaganoush
Socca Pizza Bites
Eggplant & Tomato Pesto Rolls with Coconut Tzatziki
Mini Baked Potatoes with Cashew Sour Cream & Chives
Charred Padrón Peppers with Cashew Chipotle Cream

MOCKTAILS & COCKTAILS

Sparkling Pineapple & Cayenne
Coconut, Raspberry & Mint Refresher
Passion Fruit Spritz
Watermelon & Cucumber Cooler

EASY AFTERNOON TEA

Cucumber & Lemon Butter Bean Hummus Open Sandwiches
Banana & Raisin Cake
Ginger Muffins

BIRTHDAY TEA

Peanut Butter & Honey Oat Bars
Celebration Cake
Blueberry Scones with Vanilla Coconut Cream

BEET & SWEET POTATO CHIPS

I love these. They are the most moreish little snacks and they look so beautiful, too, with their bright pink and orange coloring. They taste amazing on their own with just a sprinkling of sea salt, but they're also amazing dunked into Roast Carrot Hummus or Herby Guacamole (pages 200 and 52).

Serves 2

NUT-FREE

1 medium sweet potato, well scrubbed
2 small beets, well scrubbed
olive oil
salt

Preheat the oven to 300°F.

Using a mandoline or a very sharp knife, thinly slice the veg into rounds and lay the slices on a piece of paper towel, then press another sheet of paper towel over the top to blot them dry.

Lightly brush a couple of baking sheets with olive oil, then lay the veg slices on top, making sure they don't overlap or touch. Then pour some more oil into a small bowl and, using a pastry brush, brush oil onto each round. (This step is laborious, but it will make them so crispy and delicious in the end that it's worth taking the time to do it properly. Enjoy the moment!)

Put them in the oven and set the timer for 15 minutes. When the timer goes off, take out each sheet, and any that have crisped up nicely can be carefully plucked off and laid onto a wire rack to cool. Turn the rest over onto their other sides, return them to the oven and set the timer for another 10 minutes.

When the timer goes off again, check your sheets, and again place any that are done on the wire rack. The rest go back into the oven for another 5 minutes. When this time is up, they should all be ready, but if not keep going—checking and turning every 5 minutes—until you're satisfied.

Once your chips are all on the rack and cool, put them in a bowl and sprinkle with a little salt before serving.

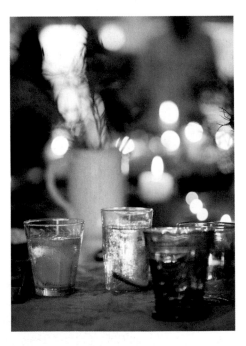

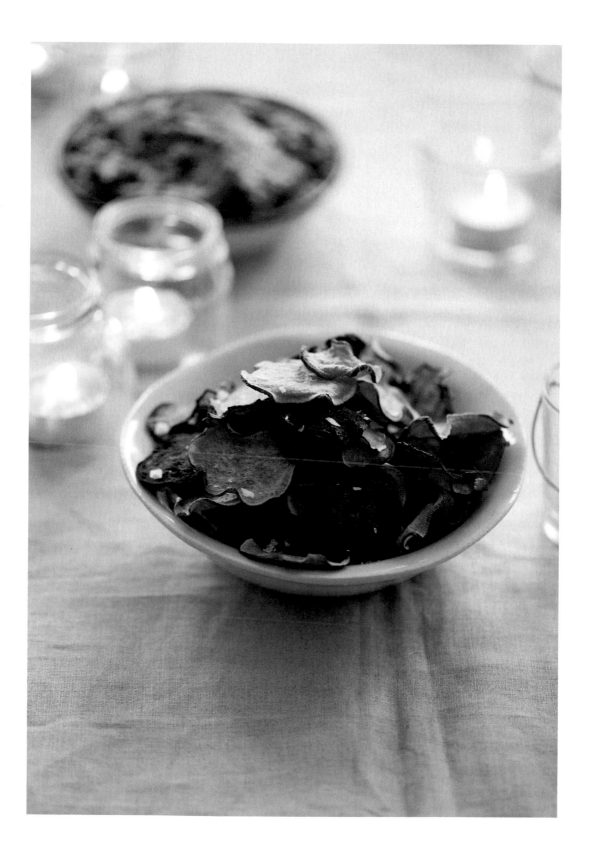

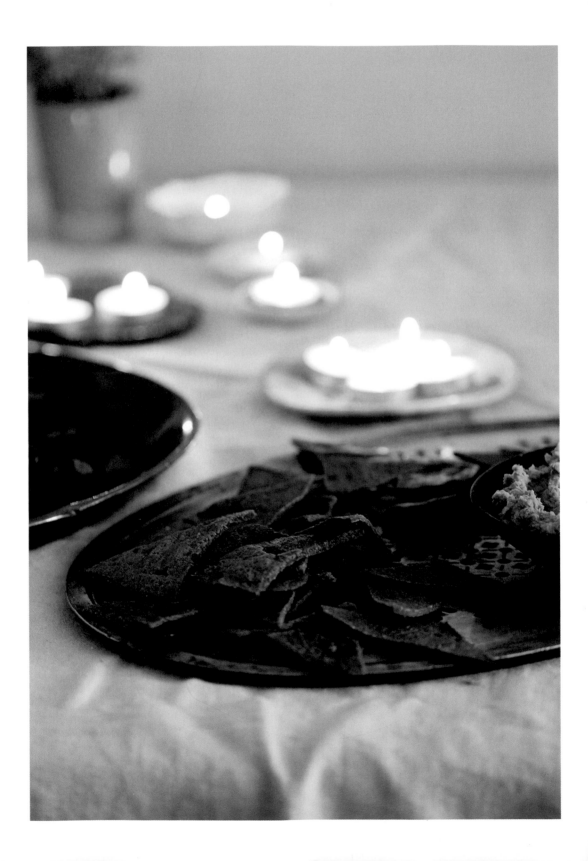

SMOKY BAKED TORTILLA CHIPS

A fantastic addition to any party, these are relatively quick to make, and it's really fun to serve home-made tortilla chips; I'm sure all your friends will be suitably impressed! Perfect with Roast Carrot Hummus (page 200), or any other dip. Be warned, they're addictive, so you may find the whole bowl is gone before your guests even arrive . . .

Serves 6–8

NUT-FREE

generous ¾ cup buckwheat flour

¾ cup cornmeal

3 tablespoons ground chia seeds (if you can't find them ground, just grind the seeds yourself at home)

2 heaping teaspoons smoked paprika

2 teaspoons chili flakes

1 teaspoon salt

1 teaspoon honey

Preheat the oven to 400°F.

Mix all the dry ingredients in a bowl. Add the honey, then pour in ½ cup plus 2 tablespoons water. Mix into a paste with a fork and set aside.

On a clean dry surface, lay down a square of parchment paper. Cut another square of parchment paper and set aside.

Wet your hands and pick up half the tortilla mixture from the bowl. Roll it in your palms until it's a nice smooth ball and drop it into the center of the parchment. Place the second sheet of parchment on top and squash the dough down gently with your hand into a disc. Take a rolling pin and roll it from the center outward to make a nice round about 8 inches across. Place on a baking sheet, leaving both sheets of parchment on. Repeat to roll the remaining dough and place on a separate baking sheet.

Put both tortillas in the oven for 10 minutes, then remove and peel off the top layers of parchment. Cut each into 8 wedges, as you would cut a pizza. (You can use a knife, but I find scissors much easier.) The tortilla will be hot, so watch you don't burn your fingers, but do it straightaway or it will become too brittle to cut. Repeat with the second tortilla.

Return the tortilla triangles to their baking sheets and bake for 5 minutes, or until they harden up. Cool on a wire rack, then serve as soon as possible.

ROAST CARROT HUMMUS

As lots of you will know by now, hummus is one of my favorite foods, and I find that all my friends and family love it, too. Everyone always gets so excited by how much better homemade hummus tastes than the store-bought versions! I make a variety of hummus almost every time I have people over, as it's such a good predinner snack, and it's so easy to throw together in no time. I especially love this carroty one, as the color is so fantastic. Once I've made my hummus, I just scoop it out of the food processor into a nice bowl and lay it out with my Smoky Baked Tortilla Chips (page 199) for everyone to enjoy when they arrive. If I want it to look more impressive, I'll drizzle it with a little olive oil, then sprinkle toasted pine nuts and smoked paprika over the top.

Makes about 4 cups

NUT-FREE

4 medium carrots (about 14 ounces), peeled

1½ teaspoons paprika

½ cup plus 2 tablespoons olive oil, plus more for drizzling

salt

3 garlic cloves, peeled

two 15-ounce cans chickpeas, drained and rinsed

3 tablespoons tahini

juice of 2 juicy lemons, or 3 if they're not very juicy

1 teaspoon ground cumin

Preheat the oven to 425°F.

Chop the carrots into quarters, then put them on a baking sheet with ½ teaspoon of the paprika, a drizzle of olive oil and a sprinkling of salt. Roast for about 40 minutes, or until soft and tender, adding the garlic cloves for the last 10 minutes. Let cool.

Meanwhile, place the chickpeas in a food processor with the ½ cup plus 2 tablespoons olive oil, the tahini, lemon juice, cumin, remaining 1 teaspoon paprika and salt to taste. Add ¼ cup water and blend until smooth and creamy.

Once the carrots and garlic have cooled, add them to the processor and finish blending. When the hummus is smooth and creamy, scoop it into a bowl and serve.

This will keep in an airtight container in the fridge for up to 7 days.

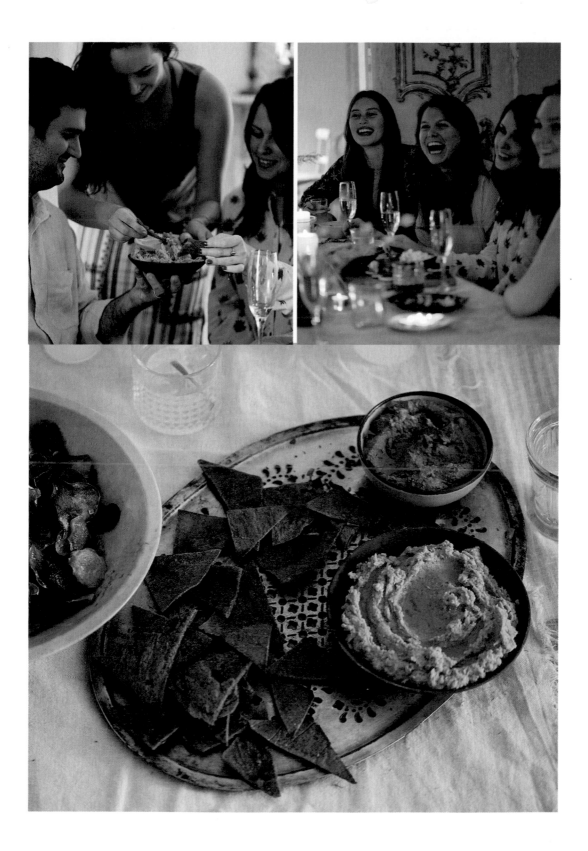

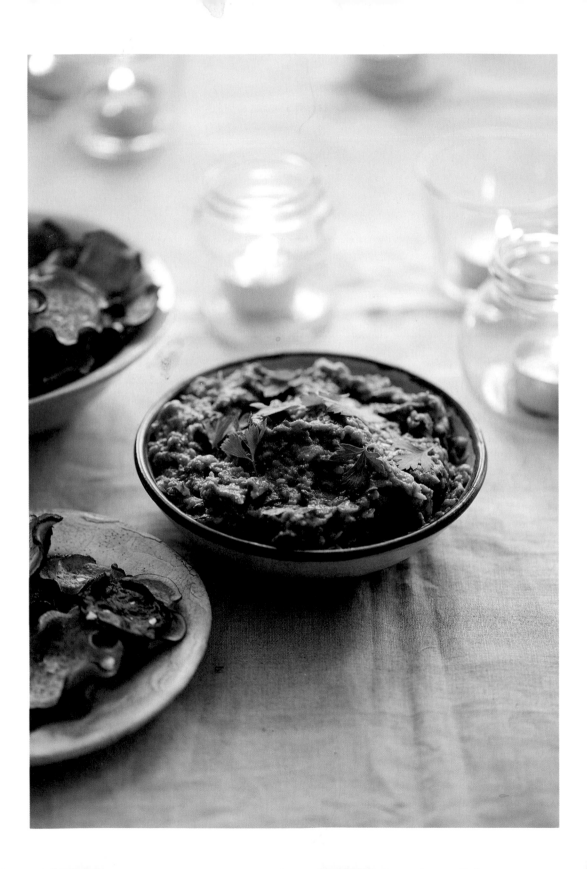

SMOKY BABAGANOUSH

One of my best-loved dips; I just love how rich and creamy this is. Chunky baked eggplant adds such a great texture, while the paprika and cayenne really liven it up and add a smoky spice to each bite. I like to serve this to friends with Smoky Baked Tortilla Chips (page 199) or crackers as a prelunch snack, or just to dollop it on the side of a grain and veggie bowl.

Makes about 3 cups

NUT-FREE

3 eggplants

1 bulb garlic

3 tablespoons olive oil, plus more for drizzling

juice of 1 lemon

1 tablespoon tahini

2 teaspoons smoked paprika

½ teaspoon ground cumin

¼ teaspoon cayenne pepper

salt and pepper

handful of fresh parsley leaves, roughly chopped

Preheat the oven to 425°F.

Prick each eggplant in a couple of places with a knife; this is essential to stop them from exploding as they bake! Put them on a baking sheet and bake for 40 minutes, turning halfway through, until their skins are blackened and the insides feel soft when pressed. Place the whole bulb of garlic, just as it is, in a square of foil, drizzle with oil, then seal the foil as though it was a little parcel (this stops it from burning) and pop it onto the baking sheet in the oven alongside the eggplants for 30 minutes.

Take the eggplants and garlic out of the oven, halve the eggplants lengthwise and let everything cool.

When they're cool enough to handle, scoop out the flesh of the eggplants into a blender. Squeeze the sticky sweet baked garlic into the blender. Add all the other ingredients except the parsley (not forgetting the 3 tablespoons of oil) and pulse a few times rather than blending completely, to avoid a totally smooth purée; you want some nice texture in there. Stir in the parsley and eat!

SOCCA PIZZA BITES

The perfect little canapé. They're so easy to make and only need a couple of really simple ingredients, plus they look fantastic. I love serving them with a dollop of the sun-dried tomato pesto below, a few chopped black olives, a sprinkling of wild arugula and a drizzle of olive oil, to heighten all the flavors. Socca is a French/Italian flatbread or pancake made from chickpea flour, and is utterly addictive.

Makes about 24

FOR THE PESTO

½ cup drained oil-packed sun-dried tomatoes

3 tablespoons pine nuts

⅓ cup fresh basil leaves

2 tablespoons olive oil

½ tablespoon apple cider vinegar

1 garlic clove, roughly chopped

salt and pepper

FOR THE PIZZAS

generous ¾ cup chickpea flour

2 teaspoons mixed dried herbs

salt and pepper

olive oil

chopped black olives, to serve

wild arugula leaves, to serve

First make the pesto by blending all the ingredients together with 2 tablespoons water in a food processor until a chunky paste forms.

In a mixing bowl, whisk together the chickpea flour and mixed herbs with ½ cup plus 2 tablespoons water, seasoning to taste, until a totally smooth batter forms. Let sit for 30 minutes for the flour to totally absorb the water.

Once you're ready to make the pizzas, heat a drizzle of olive oil in a frying pan over medium heat and, when it's hot, spoon in 1 teaspoon of the batter at a time to make each mini pizza.

Cook for 1–2 minutes, then flip and cook for another 1–2 minutes on the other side, until golden brown. Repeat this process until you have cooked all the pizza bites.

Spoon the pesto onto the pizza bases and top with the olives and a few arugula leaves to serve.

CLEVER COOKING

Try to serve these while they're still warm, as they taste even better!

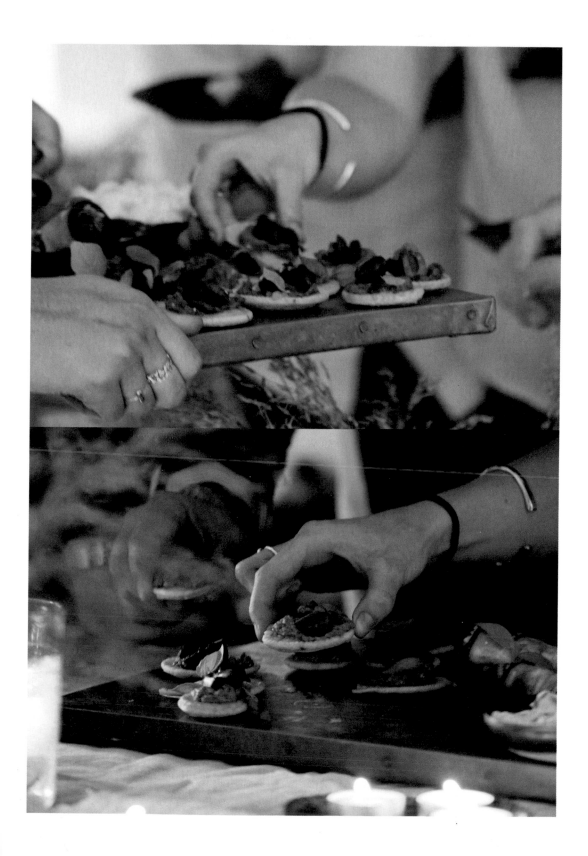

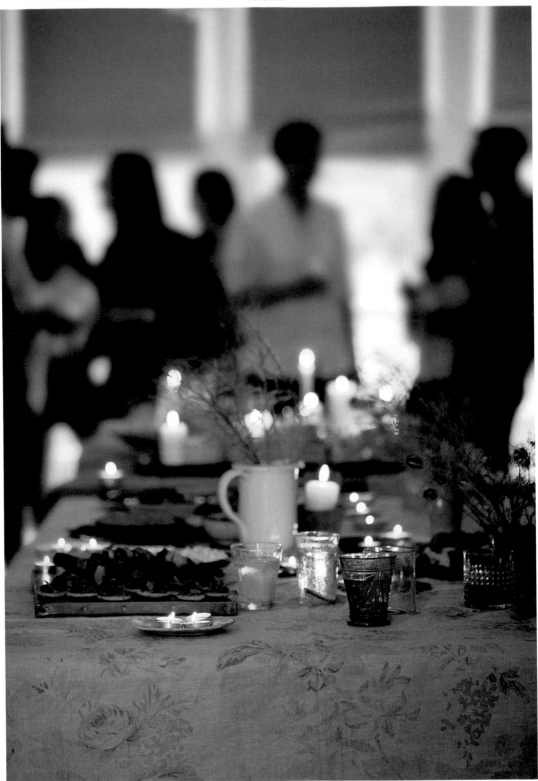

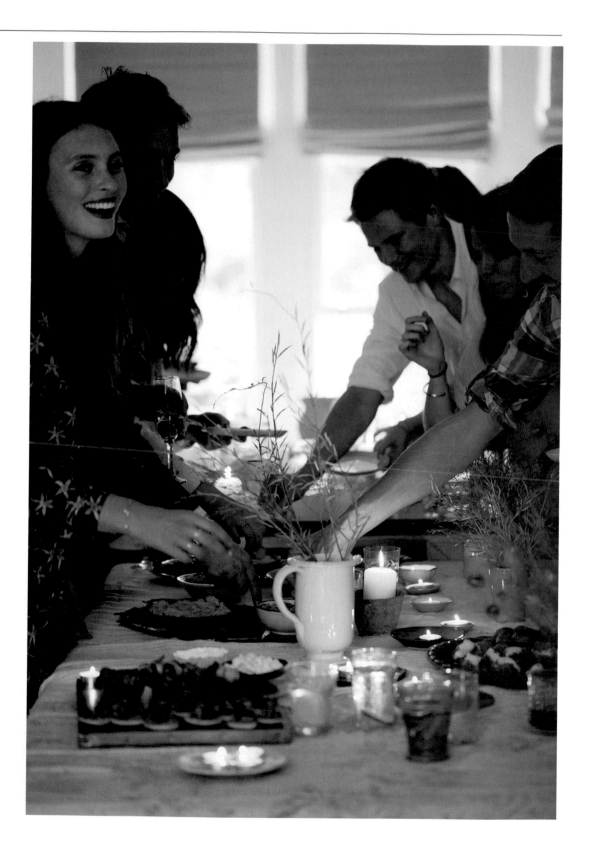

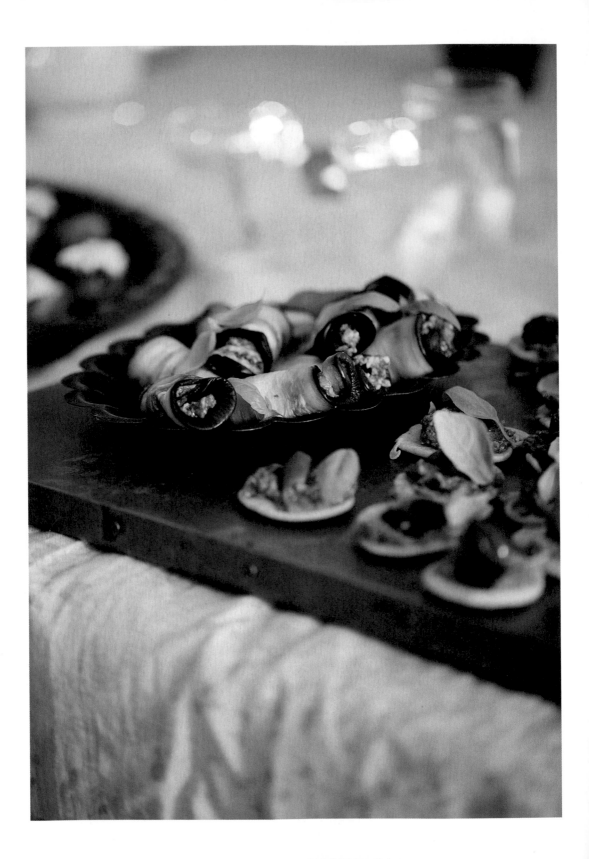

EGGPLANT & TOMATO PESTO ROLLS WITH COCONUT TZATZIKI

So great on their own, but when these rolls are dunked into the creamy mint and cucumber yogurt dip here, they become something truly special. The contrast of the hot rolls against the smooth cool dip is really amazing. These are definitely among the recipes I recommend you try first from this book; it's one of the best! The pesto is essentially the same as for Socca Pizza Bites (page 204), sharpened with lemon juice.

Makes 15 bite-size rolls

FOR THE EGGPLANT
2 large eggplants
2 tablespoons olive oil
salt

FOR THE PESTO
5 tablespoons pine nuts
one 10-ounce jar oil-packed sun-dried
    tomatoes, drained (6 ounces drained
    weight)
small handful of fresh basil
1 small garlic clove
juice of ½ lemon

FOR THE DIP
½ cucumber
leaves from a few sprigs of fresh mint
1 cup coconut yogurt
juice of 1 lemon

CLEVER COOKING
These work really well with a classic pesto, too, so if you're tight on time or don't have a food processor to blend the pesto in, you can always buy a jar and stuff the rolls with that.

Preheat the oven to 425°F.

Thinly slice the eggplants lengthwise (use a sharp knife). Drizzle a couple of large baking sheets with the olive oil and a sprinkling of salt and lay the eggplant slices evenly across them. Roast for about 20 minutes, or until soft and tender enough to roll.

Meanwhile, make the pesto. Simply place all the ingredients in a food processor and blitz until they form a chunky paste.

Let the eggplant slices cool for a few minutes, then halve each crosswise. Put 1 heaping teaspoon of pesto at the top of each, then roll them up. (You can use toothpicks to keep them together if you want.)

To make the dipping sauce, seed the cucumber by halving it lengthwise and running a teaspoon along the center. Cut it into little cubes (about ¼ inch). Finely chop the mint. Place the mint and cucumber in a bowl with the yogurt and lemon juice, season to taste and stir. Serve with the eggplant rolls.

MINI BAKED POTATOES WITH CASHEW SOUR CREAM & CHIVES

An amazing little nibble for hungry friends. These warm, salt-crusted potatoes are stuffed with a creamy cashew sour cream, then sprinkled with lots of black pepper, chives and fresh chile to make something incredibly delicious. They're perfect in the winter, hearty and comforting, and will keep everyone happy while you finish making dinner.

Serves 6

Cashew Sour Cream (page 115)
1 pound new potatoes
1 tablespoon olive oil
flaky sea salt and pepper
1 fresh red chile, seeded and chopped
1 tablespoon chopped chives

CLEVER COOKING

Serve these on a warmed sheet so that they don't get cold too quickly.

Make the Cashew Sour Cream as directed on page 115.

Preheat the oven to 410°F. Line a baking sheet with parchment paper.

Prick the potatoes with a fork, then rub them with the olive oil and sprinkle them with a generous amount of sea salt. Place them on the prepared sheet and bake for 1 hour, or until crisp on the outside and tender on the inside.

Let them cool for 10–15 minutes, until they're still warm but not boiling. Then, cut a cross in the top of each and squeeze up from the bottom to open the cut a little (use a tea towel to protect your hands from burning).

Add 1 teaspoon of the cashew sour cream to each potato, pushing it into the opening. Grind lots of black pepper over the top and sprinkle with salt, chives and chile.

Serve straightaway.

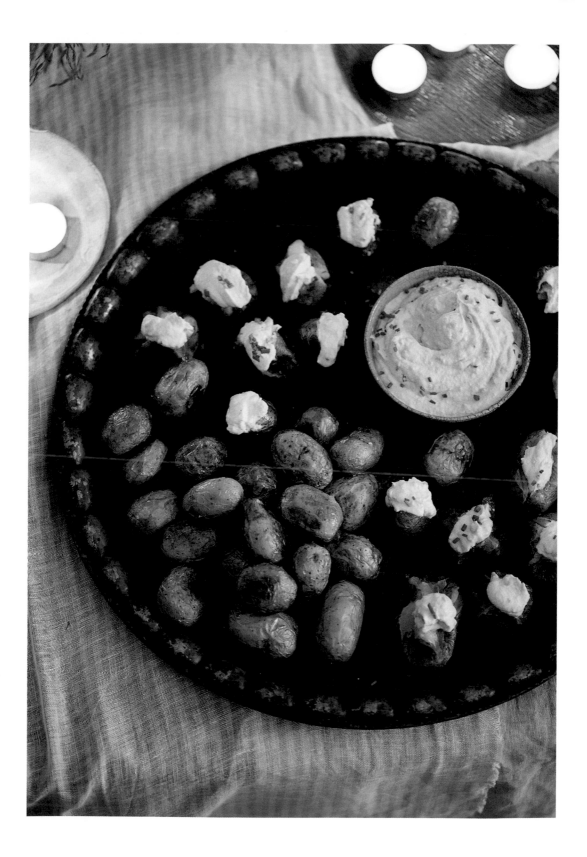

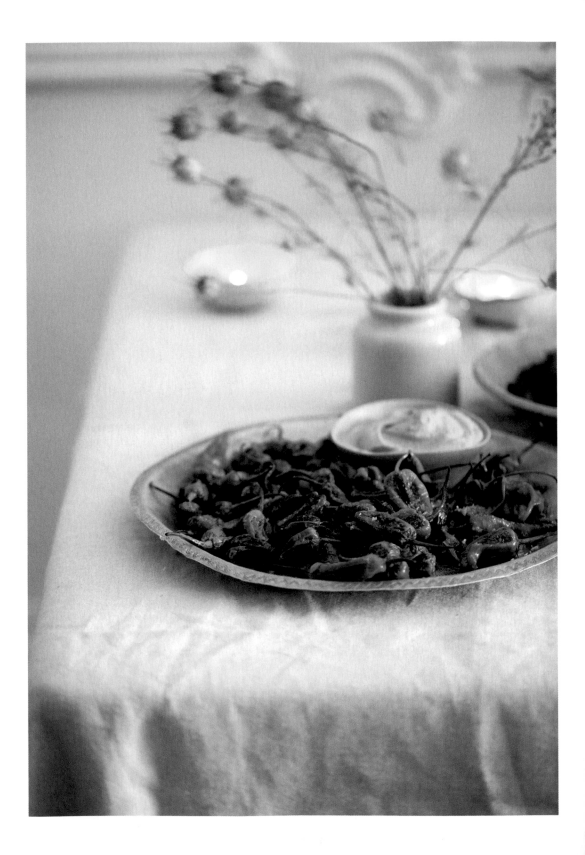

CHARRED PADRÓN PEPPERS WITH CASHEW CHIPOTLE CREAM

Padrón peppers are always one of the first things I look for on a restaurant menu; I just love them. They're so moreish, especially when they're nicely blistered and piping hot. I find they're especially good when you have something to dip them in, which is where this chipotle cream comes in. It's wonderfully smoky, with tangy hints of lemon and deeply savory sesame oil.

Makes about 1½ cups

FOR THE CHIPOTLE CREAM

1¼ cups cashews, soaked for 4 hours and drained

juice of 2 lemons

2 tablespoons apple cider vinegar

3 tablespoons olive oil

1 teaspoon toasted sesame oil

2 teaspoons chipotle powder

½ teaspoon smoked paprika

generous amount of salt

FOR THE PEPPERS

olive oil

10 ounces Padrón peppers

flaky sea salt

Place the drained cashews in a blender and add ¾ cup water. Add all the other ingredients for the chipotle cream and blend until the mixture is smooth and creamy. Scrape it into a bowl.

Heat a little olive oil in a large frying pan over medium-high heat. Add the peppers and a generous amount of sea salt and fry until they start to blister; about 10 minutes.

Serve the peppers with the chipotle cream.

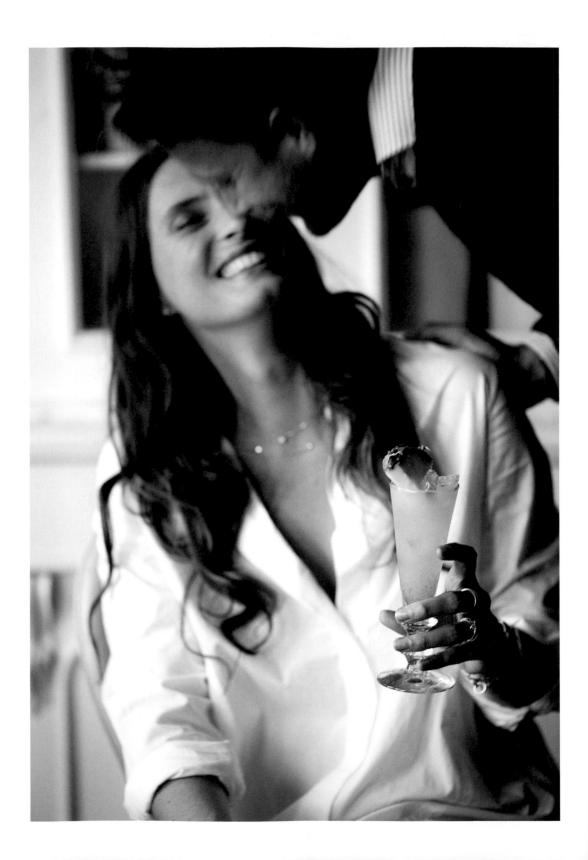

SPARKLING PINEAPPLE & CAYENNE

One of my all-time favorite drinks, this is amazingly sweet and refreshing with a subtle hint of spice from the ginger and cayenne and a little tanginess from lime juice, plus a subtle sparkle from the soda water. I like serving it in short glasses with lots of ice, a wedge of juicy pineapple and a sprinkling of more cayenne . . . it's the perfect addition to any summer party or dinner with friends. If you want to make these really fun, serve them in carved-out pineapples! You can make this in a juicer or a blender.

Serves 3

1 pineapple
1 inch fresh ginger, peeled
1⅔ cups club soda
juice of ½ lime
2 teaspoons maple syrup
generous pinch of cayenne pepper, to taste
    (I like quite a lot, about 3 pinches), plus
    more to serve
dash of your favorite spirit (optional)
ice cubes

Cut the hard skin off the pineapple, then cut a small slice off the top for garnishing later. Put the rest of the pineapple through a juicer with the ginger, passing the ginger through toward the start of the operation, to get the most flavor out of it.

Pour the juice through a sieve into a pitcher, to make sure it's really smooth.

Pour the club soda into the pitcher, then add the lime juice, maple syrup and cayenne to taste, along with the spirit, if you like. Stir well.

Fill 3 short glasses with ice and pour the drink into each. Sprinkle with a pinch more cayenne and add a wedge of pineapple from the reserved slice to the side of the glass.

CLEVER COOKING
If you don't have a juicer, put the ginger and pineapple in your blender instead, then strain the blended mixture through a sieve to make it smooth.

COCONUT, RASPBERRY & MINT REFRESHER

This is a wonderfully refreshing drink made from cooling coconut water, lime juice and maple syrup, stirred with fresh mint, cucumber slices and raspberries. It looks beautiful with the mix of greens and pinks, so a big pitcher of this is a lovely addition to any table. Measure out the coconut water using the glasses in which you will be serving it.

Serves 3

¼ cucumber
1 ounce sprigs of fresh mint
2½ glasses of coconut water, preferably
    raw and unpasteurized
juice of 2 limes
2 teaspoons maple syrup
6 tablespoons raspberries
ice cubes
dash of your favorite spirit (optional)

Thinly slice the cucumber and tear the mint leaves off their stems. Keep the leaves and discard the stems.

Pour the coconut water into a pitcher with the lime juice and maple syrup. Stir well, then add the cucumber slices, mint leaves and raspberries.

Let the drink sit in the fridge for at least 30 minutes, so that the flavors can be absorbed into the water.

Once you're ready to serve, add ice cubes to 3 glasses and stir your spirit (if using) into the pitcher.

Pour the mix into the glasses, trying to get the mint, cucumber and raspberries evenly distributed among them.

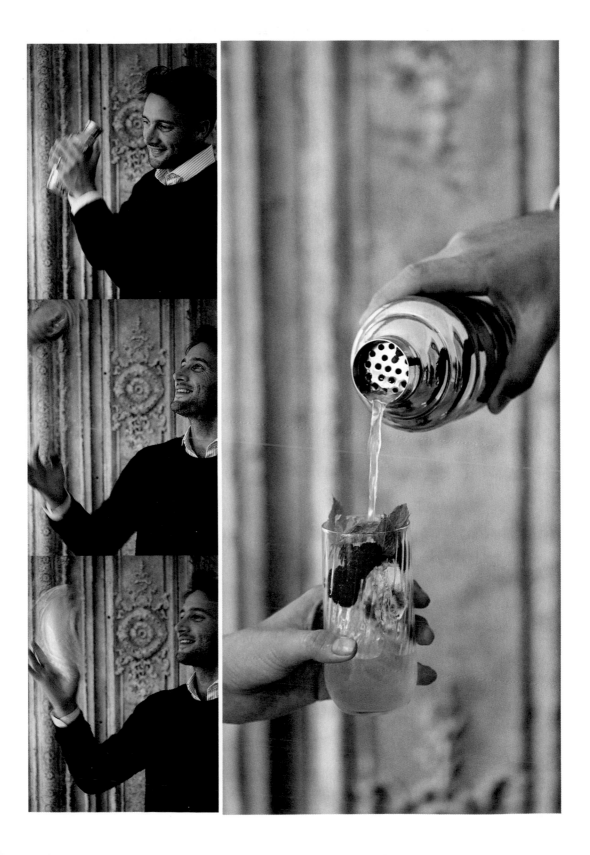

PASSION FRUIT SPRITZ

This is so lovely and I'm sure will be a big hit with all your friends. The tropical mix tastes amazing with a little vanilla powder and sparkling water. Try serving this with the Mexican Fiesta (pages 110–117); they're perfect together.

Serves 2

3 passion fruits, halved
½ mango, peeled and pitted
juice of ½ lime
½ teaspoon vanilla powder
about 1 cup sparkling water
ice cubes

Put the passion fruit pulp through a juicer and add the mango. Add the lime juice and vanilla powder and give it a good stir.

Pour into 2 short glasses, then top up both with sparkling water and a few ice cubes.

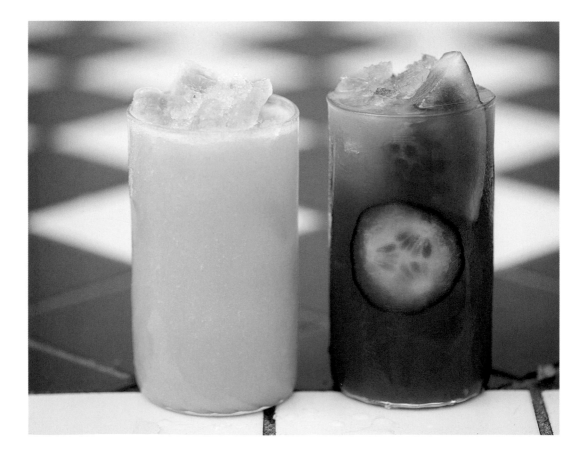

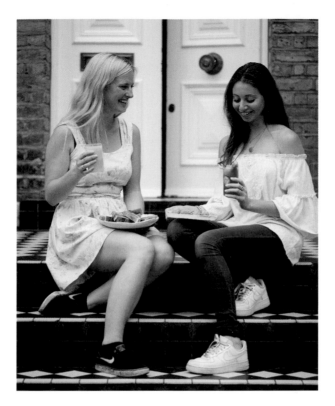

WATERMELON & CUCUMBER COOLER

This is a great summer drink, sweet and refreshing with a lovely mix of watermelon, cucumber and strawberries. We served this at our wedding and everyone loved it! It's simple and quick and very unfussy; it just needs five minutes to make, so you and your guests will have a delicious drink in no time.

Serves 2

½ cucumber
14 ounces watermelon flesh, rind cut off, and seeded
5 strawberries, hulled
2 teaspoons maple syrup (optional)
dash of your favorite spirit (optional)
ice cubes

Juice the cucumber.

Pour the juice into a blender with the watermelon, strawberries and maple syrup (if using). Blend until smooth. Pour through a sieve into a pitcher to remove any lumps, then spoon any excess foam off the top.

Stir in the spirit, if using.

Add ice cubes to 2 tall glasses and pour the drink in.

CUCUMBER & LEMON BUTTER BEAN HUMMUS OPEN SANDWICHES

These simple little sandwiches are a lovely addition to any afternoon tea or snack time. The creamy, lemony hummus tastes amazing topped with crunchy slices of cucumber, a sprinkling of lemon zest and lots of black pepper. I often make these as an afternoon snack and keep the rest of the hummus in the fridge to use throughout the week, dolloped on the side of other meals.

Makes 12

NUT-FREE

FOR THE HUMMUS

one 15-ounce can butter beans (or lima
    beans), drained and rinsed
1 garlic clove
juice of 1½ lemons
2 tablespoons olive oil
1 tablespoon tahini
2 teaspoons ground cumin
salt to taste

FOR THE SANDWICHES

3 slices square bread (I use rye bread)
½ cucumber, thinly sliced
finely grated zest and juice of
    1 unwaxed lemon
flaky sea salt and pepper

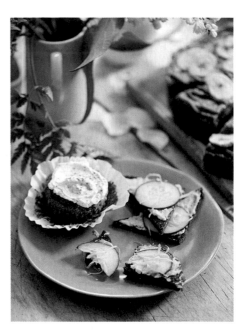

First make the hummus. Simply place everything in a food processor and blend until smooth and creamy.

Either toast the bread, if you want it crunchy, or leave it (I find rye bread and most gluten-free breads are nicer toasted).

Spread a thick layer of hummus over the bread or toast, then add crunchy slices of cucumber. Sprinkle with lemon zest to add color and texture, then squeeze a little lemon juice on each, sprinkle with sea salt and grind over lots of pepper. Cut each into quarters to serve.

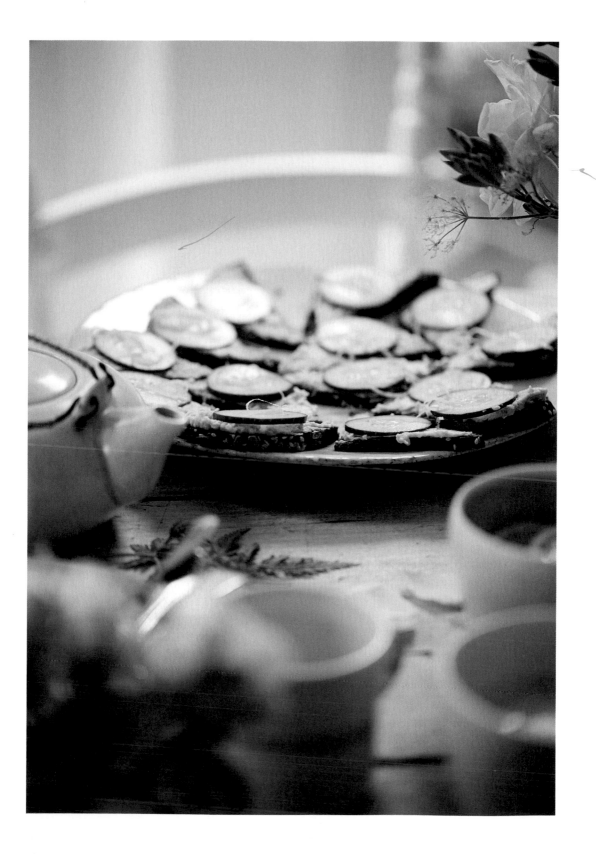

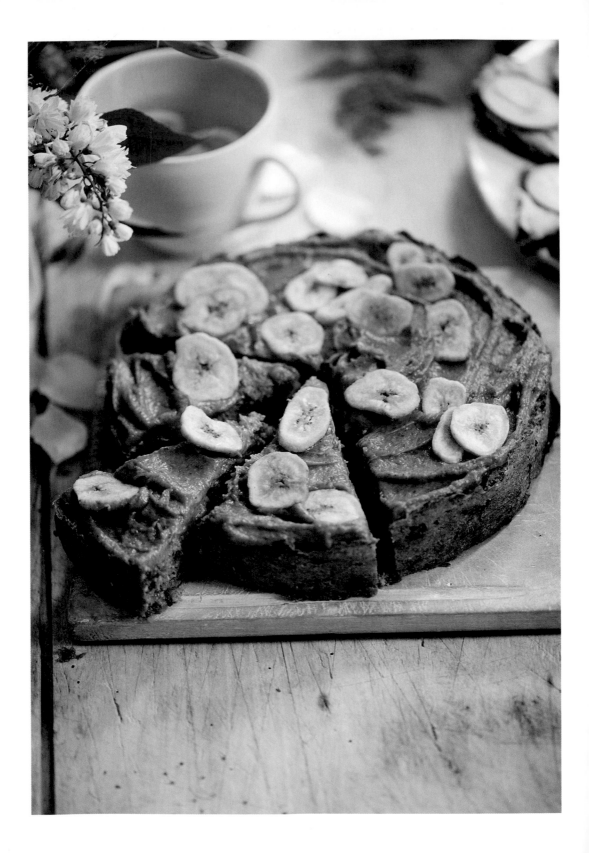

BANANA & RAISIN CAKE

This is one of my favorite cakes; it's such a great treat to serve your friends and family. It's soft and light, with juicy bites of raisins and sweet hints of coconut. It's a pretty easy recipe, plus it's the best way to use up old bananas, which I always seem to have in my kitchen! Your guests will absolutely love feasting on slices of this alongside Ginger Muffins and Cucumber & Lemon Butter Bean Hummus Open Sandwiches (pages 224 and 220); together they make a really wonderful afternoon tea.

Makes one 9-inch cake

FOR THE CAKE

2 tablespoons coconut oil,
   plus more for the pan
4 overripe bananas
3¾ cups rolled oats
12½ ounces apple purée (page 23)
1 tablespoon ground cinnamon
2 teaspoons vanilla powder
¼ cup coconut sugar
scant 1 cup raisins
2 tablespoons chia seeds

FOR THE ICING

2 overripe bananas
4 medjool dates, pitted
1 teaspoon vanilla powder
2 tablespoons coconut oil
2 tablespoons almond butter
½ teaspoon ground cinnamon,
   plus more to serve
banana chips, to decorate (optional)

Preheat the oven to 400°F. Use coconut oil to oil 9-inch round cake pan, or line it with a round of parchment paper.

Mash the bananas with a fork in a large bowl. Grind the oats into a flour in a food processor. Melt the 2 tablespoons of coconut oil in a small saucepan. Add the oat flour and coconut oil to the bananas along with the remaining cake ingredients. Scrape the batter into the prepared pan.

Bake for 50 minutes, or until a knife poked in comes out clean. Let cool in the pan for 30 minutes to finish setting.

Meanwhile, make the icing. Simply blend all the ingredients (except the banana chips) until totally smooth, then put the icing in the fridge to set for 10–20 minutes, while the cake cools.

When the cake is totally cool, remove it from the pan and spread the icing over the top. Decorate with banana chips, if you like, and sprinkle with cinnamon.

GINGER MUFFINS

I'm a big ginger fan. I love the warming sensation it brings to any dish, especially when combined with vanilla, cinnamon and nutmeg, as it is here. The spices work so well in these muffins, creating a really uplifting little afternoon snack. The icing is totally optional, so if you want something that's easy to carry around, I'd skip it as it can get messy in a lunch box. But if you're staying put, then absolutely add it, as it heightens the deliciousness and adds a smooth, creamy texture to the oaty muffins.

Makes 12

FOR THE MUFFINS

1 cup coconut yogurt
2 tablespoons psyllium husk (from natural foods stores or online)
1⅓ cups brown rice flour
6 tablespoons coconut flour
¾ cup plus 2 tablespoons rolled oats
½ cup coconut sugar
2 teaspoons ground cinnamon
2 teaspoons vanilla powder
1 teaspoon ground nutmeg
1 tablespoon ground ginger
2 overripe bananas, mashed
2 tablespoons coconut oil, melted
2 tablespoons maple syrup

FOR THE ICING

1 cup coconut yogurt
1 teaspoon ground ginger, plus more to serve (optional)
2 tablespoons maple syrup
ground ginger or cinnamon (optional)

Preheat the oven to 400°F. Line 12 cups of a muffin pan with paper liners.

Make the muffin batter. Pour the yogurt into a large bowl. Make a psyllium husk "egg" (this helps the batter stick together): place the husk in a small bowl or mug with ¼ cup water and give it a mix. Pour into the yogurt and whisk thoroughly to combine.

Add the dry ingredients, then stir in ⅔ cup water. Stir in the bananas, coconut oil and maple syrup and mix until it forms quite a stiff batter. Spoon the batter evenly into the muffin cups.

Bake for 40 minutes. Let cool completely in the pan before icing (or the icing will melt).

To make the icing, simply mix all the ingredients together in a bowl and let it sit in the fridge for the last few minutes of the muffins cooling.

Ice each muffin and sprinkle with ground ginger or cinnamon before serving, if you like.

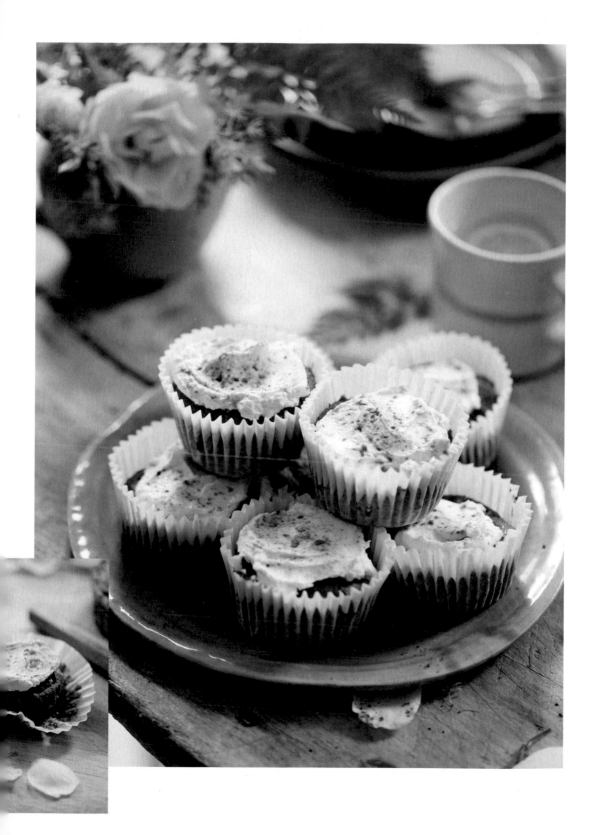

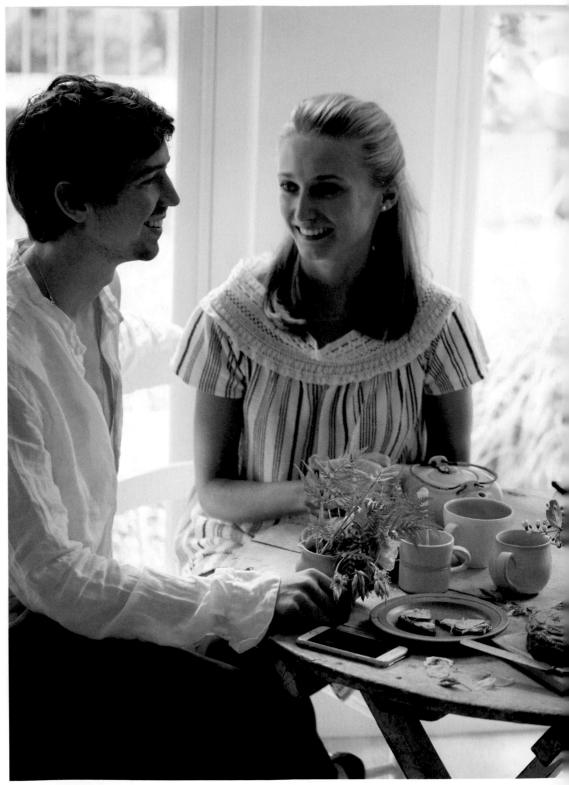

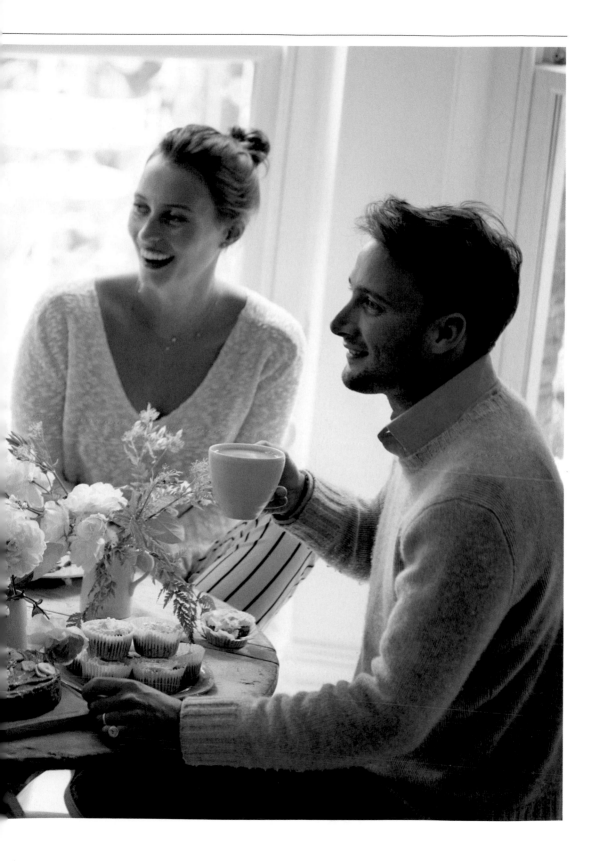

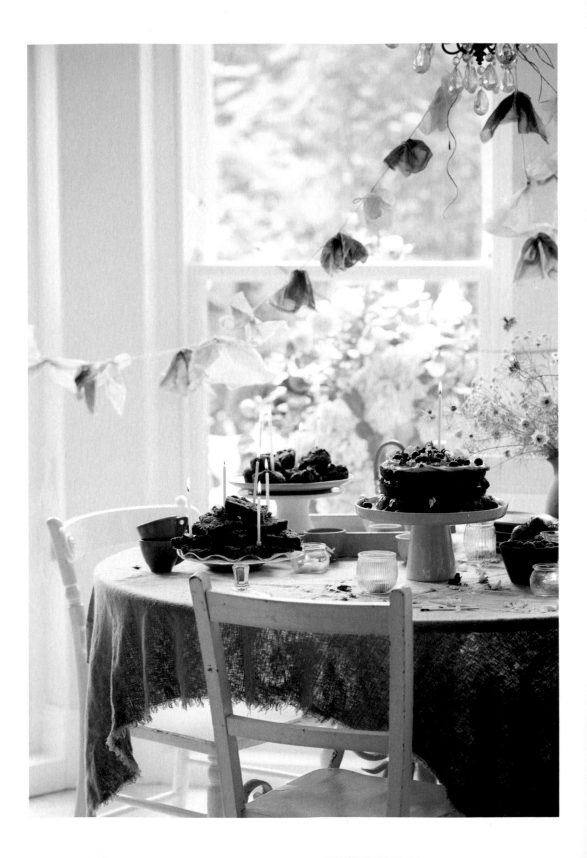

PEANUT BUTTER & HONEY OAT BARS

These are so moreish; I always get through a batch of them far too quickly! The mix of banana and peanut butter makes each bite soft and gooey, while the raisins, coconut oil and honey give a deliciously sweet taste; although, as there are only four spoons of honey across the whole batch, they're not overly sweet, which means they also work really well as an on-the-go breakfast.

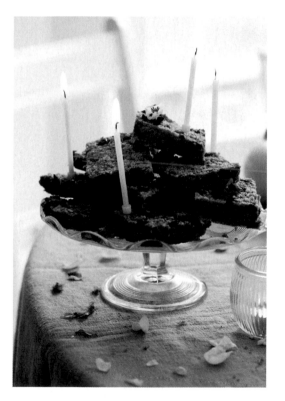

Makes 12

3 tablespoons coconut oil, plus more
    for the pan
4 overripe bananas
¼ cup honey
¼ cup crunchy peanut butter,
    or any other nut butter
1¼ cups raisins
3¾ cups rolled oats

Preheat the oven to 400°F. Oil an 8-inch square brownie pan with coconut oil, or line with parchment paper.

Mash the bananas with a fork in a bowl. Mix in the 3 tablespoons coconut oil and all the other ingredients. Pour the mixture into the prepared pan.

Bake for 30–35 minutes, until golden brown. Let sit for at least 15 minutes in the pan to finish setting. Once cool, cut into 12 bars and enjoy!

CELEBRATION CAKE

If you've got a birthday or a special event coming up that needs a sweet, indulgent cake to mark it, then this is for you. It looks incredibly impressive and decadent with its layers of vanilla and almond sponge cake layered with blueberry jam and caramel icing, then finished with coconut icing on top. The triple-layered effect makes it visually stunning, while the three different icings mean it's delicious. I tend to always go for chocolatey cakes, so this is a really nice change; and losing the chocolate also makes it feel a little lighter, so you can enjoy an extra few bites . . . or even another slice!

Serves 8–10

FOR THE CAKE

4½ tablespoons coconut oil, plus more
    for the pans
3 tablespoons chia seeds
2 teaspoons apple cider vinegar
1½ cups almond milk
1½ cups maple syrup
3 tablespoons vanilla powder
2½ cups stone-ground polenta (I like Biona
    Organic Polenta Bramata)
4¼ cups almond meal
¼ cup arrowroot powder

FOR THE BLUEBERRY JAM

1¾ cups blueberries
1 tablespoon maple syrup
2 tablespoons chia seeds

FOR THE CARAMEL ICING

10 medjool dates, pitted
3 tablespoons almond milk
¼ cup cashew butter
pinch of salt

FOR THE COCONUT ICING

3 tablespoons cashew butter
1 cup coconut yogurt
3 tablespoons coconut sugar
½ teaspoon vanilla powder

TO DECORATE
blueberries
coconut sugar
coconut chips

Preheat the oven to 380°F. Oil three 8-inch round cake pans, or line with rounds of parchment paper. Put the chia into a mug with ½ cup water. Leave for 20 minutes until the seeds expand and form a gel. Gently melt the 4½ tablespoons coconut oil.

In a large bowl, mix all the cake ingredients, including the chia and coconut oil. Stir until smooth. Divide among the prepared pans and bake for 35–40 minutes, until golden; a knife poked in should come out clean. Let the cakes cool in the pans.

Meanwhile, over medium heat, heat the ingredients for the jam in a pan for about 10 minutes, or until a thick sticky jam forms, then set aside to cool. For the caramel icing, put all the ingredients in a food processor. Blend until smooth. For the coconut icing, blend the ingredients together (or if your cashew butter isn't too solid, just stir them). Chill to set a bit.

Remove the cakes from the pans and place one layer on a plate. Thickly spread jam on

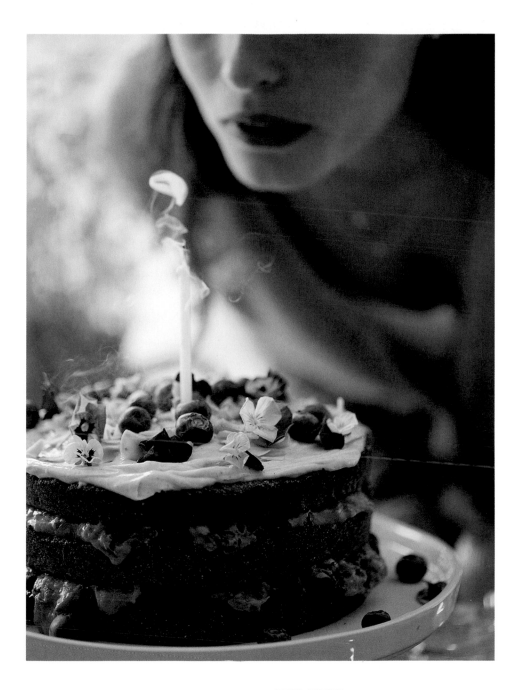

the layer (with a little caramel icing, if you like). Add a second layer and spread with the caramel icing. Put the last layer on top and spread with coconut icing. Decorate with blueberries, a sprinkling of coconut sugar and coconut chips. Enjoy!

CLEVER COOKING

Don't make the layers of the cake too thick. You want them to be an inch or so deep; any more and the cake may topple, plus it will be hard to eat!

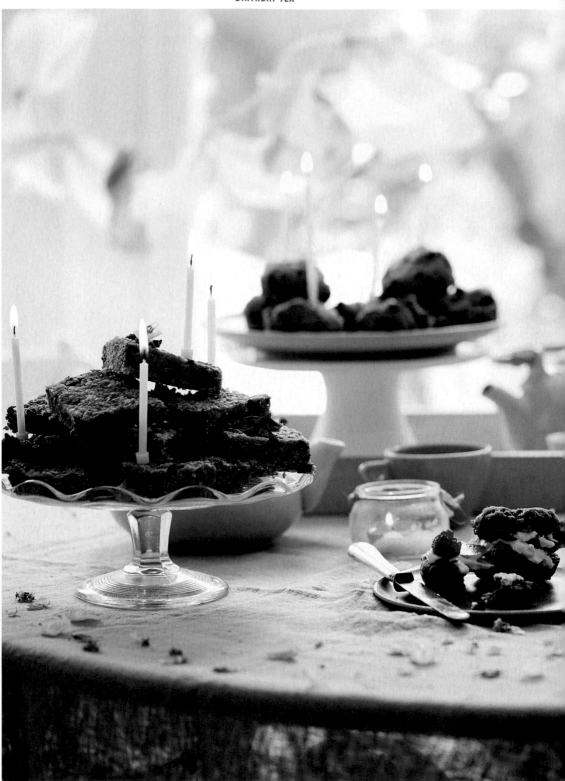

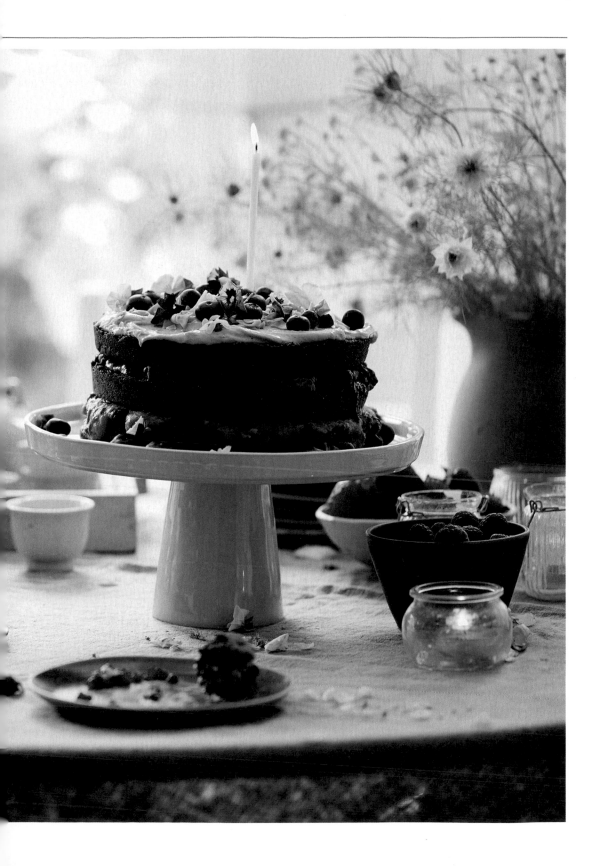

BLUEBERRY SCONES WITH VANILLA COCONUT CREAM

Scones always feel like a pretty vital part of an afternoon tea—they're just so quintessentially British—so I had to include them in this menu. These are delicious, but not overly sweet, which is refreshing if you're serving them with oat bars and cake (pages 229 and 230)! The versatile vanilla cream works with most cakes or desserts.

Makes 10

3 heaping tablespoons cold coconut oil,
   plus more for the muffin tin (optional)
2⅓ cups brown rice flour
6 tablespoons coconut sugar
2 teaspoons arrowroot powder
1 tablespoon vanilla powder
2 teaspoons ground cinnamon
1 teaspoon baking powder
pinch of salt
generous ½ cup almond milk (or oat milk or
   other plant-based milk if you prefer)
finely grated zest of 1 unwaxed lemon,
   plus the juice of ½ lemon
1 tablespoon maple syrup
1 cup blueberries
½ cup raisins

VANILLA CREAM
1 cup coconut yogurt
1 teaspoon vanilla powder
1 tablespoon light honey

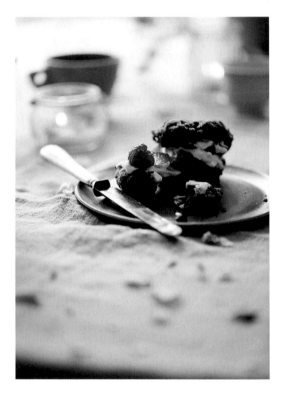

Preheat the oven to 400°F. Oil 10 cups of a muffin tin with coconut oil.

In a bowl, stir the dry ingredients together (not the blueberries or raisins) so they're well and truly mixed.

Add the 3 tablespoons of cold coconut oil and use your hands to rub it in, lifting your hands into the air over the bowl and rubbing with your fingertips, until the mixture starts to resemble breadcrumbs.

Pour in the almond milk, lemon zest and juice and maple syrup and bring it all together, kneading it in the bowl. Work in the blueberries and raisins.

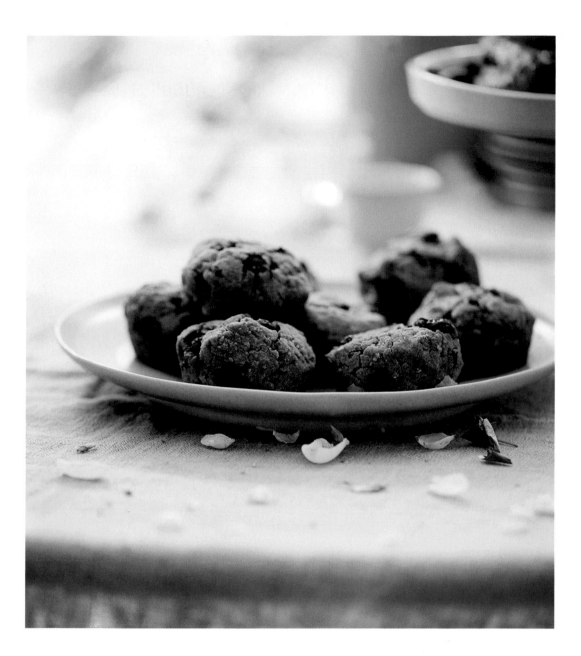

Dividing evenly, scoop the mixture into the 10 muffin cups, smoothing down the top of the scone with the back of a spoon.

Pop them in the oven for 25 minutes, or until golden brown, but check on them after 20 minutes. Remove from the oven and let cool.

Meanwhile, in a bowl, whisk together all the ingredients for the vanilla cream. Cover and keep in the fridge until ready to use. Serve the scones with the cream, adding fresh berries, if you like.

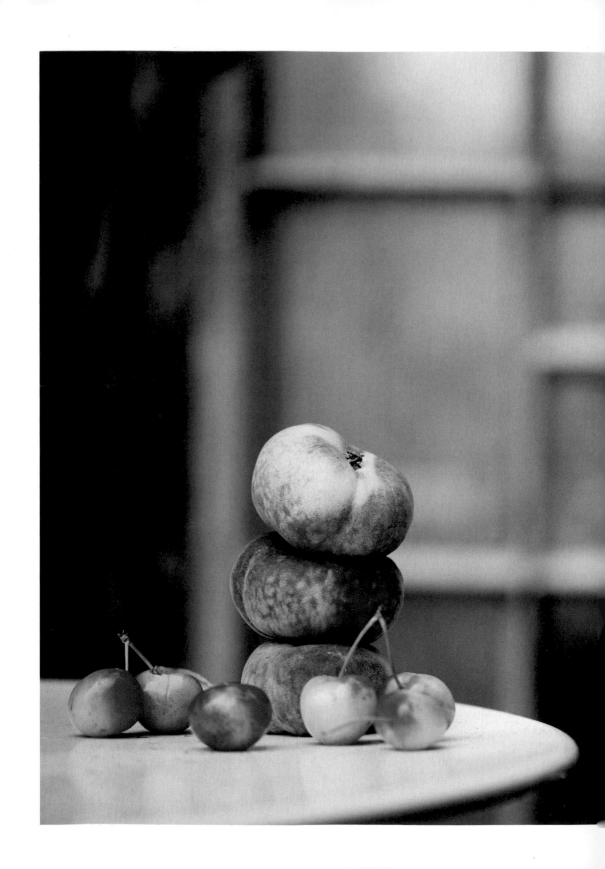

SWEETS

THE BEST WAY TO END A MEAL!

WATERMELON & MINT GRANITA

A wonderfully light, refreshing dessert that requires only three simple ingredients. It's ideal for warm summer nights with friends, especially alongside a lovely cocktail or mocktail (pages 214–219). I think it's the perfect finish to my garden party supper of Marinated Cauliflower Steaks with Chile Quinoa and Sun-Dried Tomato & Butter Bean Hummus (pages 134 and 137).

Serves 4

NUT-FREE

¾ ounce fresh mint sprigs, plus more
   to serve (optional)
about 1 pound watermelon
1 tablespoon honey

Place the mint leaves into a measuring cup and pour over ⅔ cup just-boiled water. Give it a stir and let it steep for 10 minutes.

Meanwhile, cut the rind off the watermelon and discard it. Slice up the flesh, making sure you remove all the seeds. Put the watermelon chunks into a food processor and whizz up until it's all liquid.

Remove the mint leaves from the water and discard, then stir the honey into the water until it dissolves. Stir the mint-infused honey water and puréed watermelon together, pour into a large, lidded freezer-safe container, put the lid on and put it in the freezer.

After 1 hour, remove from the freezer. Scrape off any frozen bits around the sides and mix in with the rest of the liquid, then return it to the freezer. Keep doing this every hour until you have lovely icy flakes, which you can then tumble into glasses to serve. Garnish with mint leaves, if you like.

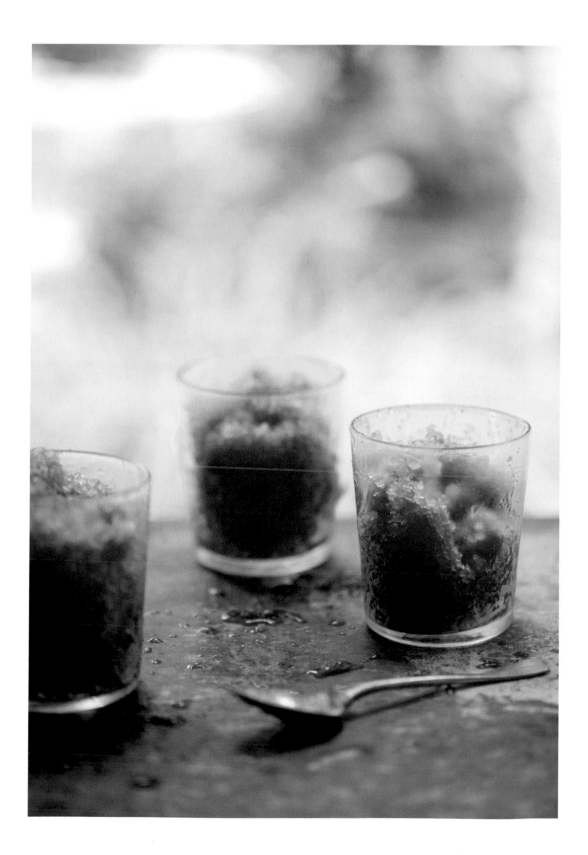

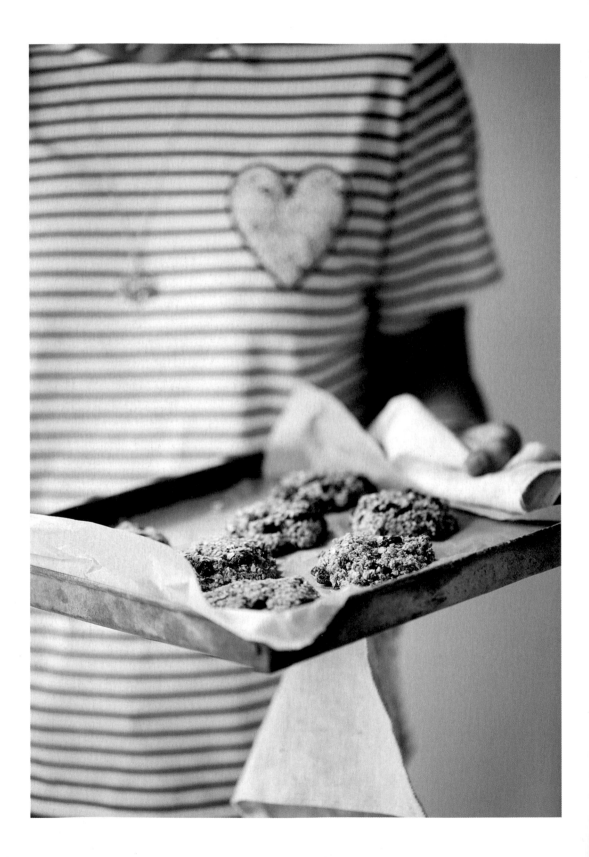

ORANGE & CARDAMOM COOKIES

These are a great staple to have in the house. They're not especially indulgent or impressive, instead they're moreish little oaty bites that satisfy an afternoon sweet tooth or a postdinner snack attack. The mix of orange, lemon, cardamom and cinnamon flavors them so nicely, while the honey and raisins add a perfect sweetness.

Makes 10–12

3–5 cardamom pods, to taste (depending on how strong you want the flavor)

3¾ cups rolled oats

6 tablespoons honey

finely grated zest of 1 unwaxed lemon, plus juice of ½ lemon

finely grated zest of 1 unwaxed orange, plus juice of ½ orange

2 tablespoons chia seeds

3 tablespoons coconut oil, melted

2 teaspoons ground cinnamon

6 tablespoons plant-based milk

¼ cup raisins

Preheat the oven to 400°F. Line a baking sheet with parchment paper.

Use the flat side of a knife to crush the cardamom pods. Once each opens, take the seeds out and grind with a mortar and pestle.

Place 2½ cups of the oats in a food processor and whizz for 30 seconds or so, until they form a flour.

Place the ground cardamom, ground oats and remaining 1¼ cups whole oats in a large bowl. Add all the remaining ingredients and stir well until a nice sticky mixture forms. It should be damp, rather than wet or runny.

Scoop 1 tablespoon of the mixture into your hand, roll it into a ball, then place it on the prepared sheet and flatten it down. Repeat to make 10–12 cookies.

Bake for 20–25 minutes, until golden brown. Let cool completely on the baking sheet, so they firm up, then serve.

CLEVER COOKING

Always zest citrus fruit before juicing it, as once you've taken the juice out it's almost impossible to zest the fruit shells.

MIX IT UP

Try smothering the cookies with a thick layer of almond butter and eating them as an afternoon snack . . . it's amazing!

PAN-FRIED CARDAMOM & HONEY APPLES

A lovely warming dessert, ideal if you want something sweet to end your meal but don't fancy spending ages chopping and prepping, or if you're keen to finish with something light. I love this served with coconut yogurt, a sprinkling of toasted nuts and sunflower seeds and a little drizzle of honey. Try making extra, so you can enjoy the leftovers as a treat with your oatmeal the next morning!

Serves 4

1 tablespoon coconut oil
1½ teaspoons ground cardamom
1½ teaspoons ground cinnamon
2 tablespoons honey
4 apples, cut into wedges

Melt the coconut oil in a large frying pan, then add the spices and honey and stir to mix. Drop in the apple chunks.

Cook everything for about 10 minutes, or until the apples are soft.

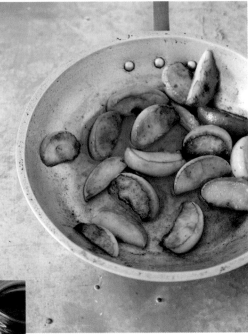

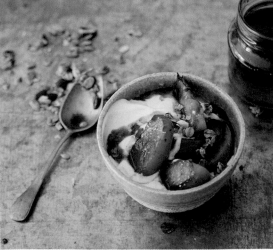

CLEVER COOKING

For this recipe, make sure you use preground cardamom rather than the seeds of cardamom pods, as you need a superfine texture. (You can grind your own seeds, but you'll have to make sure they're properly ground into a powder, then sifted, rather than just being roughly crushed.)

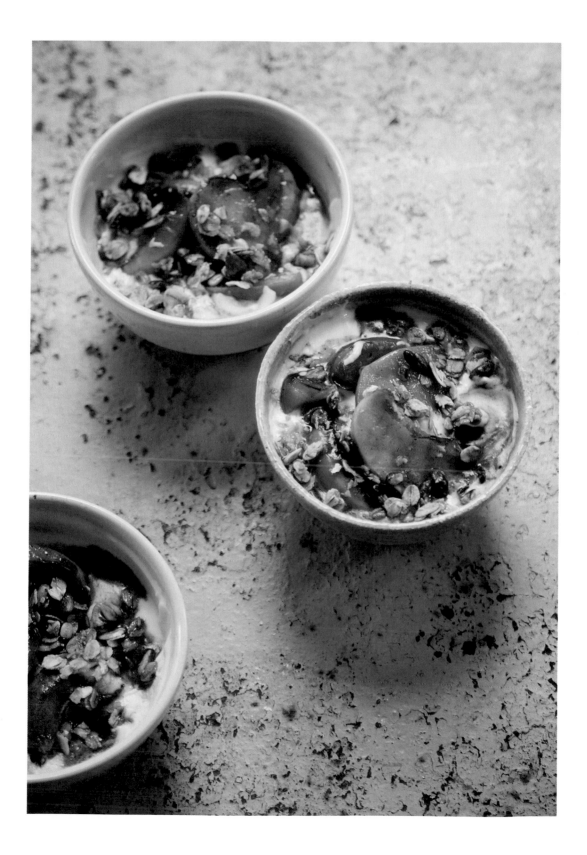

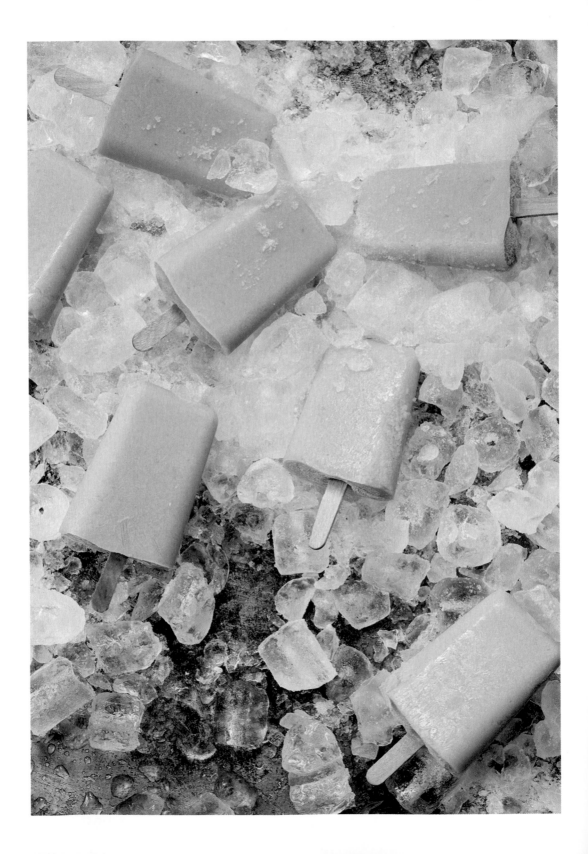

COCONUT & MANGO ICE POPS

These are a summer staple. They're unbelievably simple to make; all you need to do is blend four ingredients together and then leave them in the freezer until you're ready to enjoy. I love knowing I have a little stash of these, too, so that as soon as the weather heats up I can cool off with one of them. They make a great end to a curry.

Makes 6

1 banana (about 7 ounces), roughly chopped
1 mango (about 11 ounces), roughly chopped
generous ¾ cup coconut milk
1 tablespoon honey

Place all the ingredients in a blender and blend for 1 minute until smooth.

Pour into ice-pop molds and freeze for about 5 hours to set.

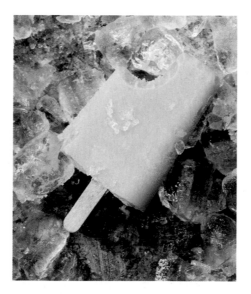

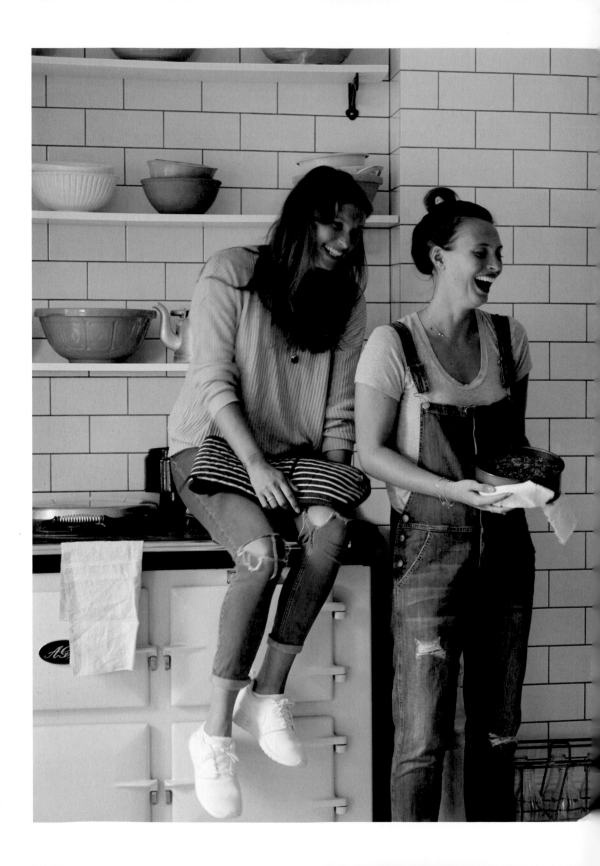

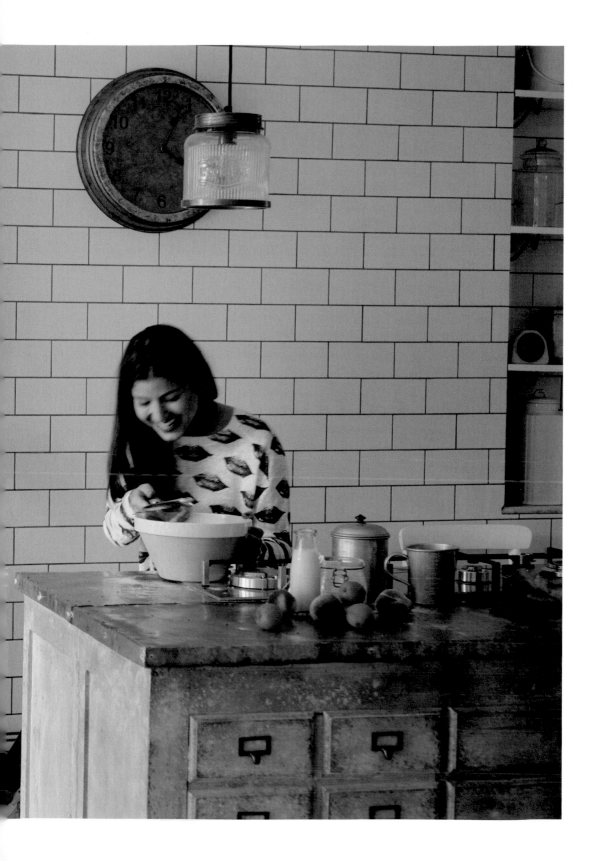

SALTED MACA & TAHINI FUDGE

Definitely one of my favorite recipes in this book, this is completely delicious and utterly addictive. The first time I made this fudge I couldn't stop thinking about it for weeks afterward. I would literally dream of it, so I had to keep making it time and again to satisfy my cravings! This is a great treat option if you just want a little sweet bite, rather than a big dessert; or eat it with tea and coffee afterward if you want both!

Makes 16–20 pieces

1½ cups cashews

1½ teaspoons vanilla powder

6 medjool dates, pitted

2 tablespoons maca powder

3 tablespoons coconut sugar

3 tablespoons tahini

flaky sea salt

Preheat the oven to 425°F. Line a loaf pan with plastic wrap.

Spread the cashews on a baking sheet and roast on the top rack for 5 minutes, or until they start to turn golden brown. Remove from the oven and let cool. Place them in a powerful food processor with the vanilla powder and blend until they form a creamy cashew butter.

Add the dates, maca, coconut sugar and tahini to the food processor and blend for another 5 minutes, or until the dates have broken down and the mixture is smooth (it may be a bit crumbly but that's OK!).

Spoon the mixture into the prepared pan, pressing it down with a spatula to make it even. Sprinkle the top with sea salt and place in the freezer for 2 hours to firm up.

Store the fudge in the freezer, taking it out 30 minutes prior to serving to soften a little bit before eating. Enjoy!

CLEVER COOKING

These look super cute and are easier to take with you out and about if you wrap them individually in twists of wax paper.

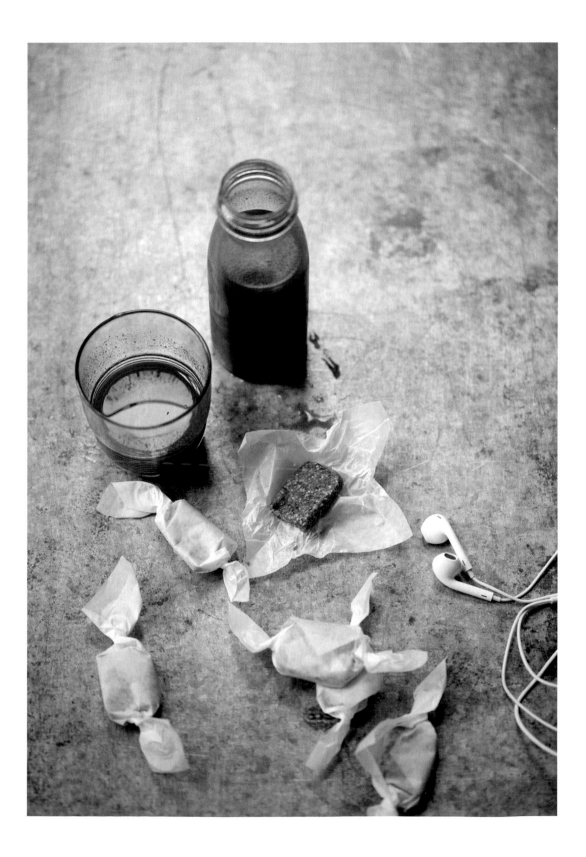

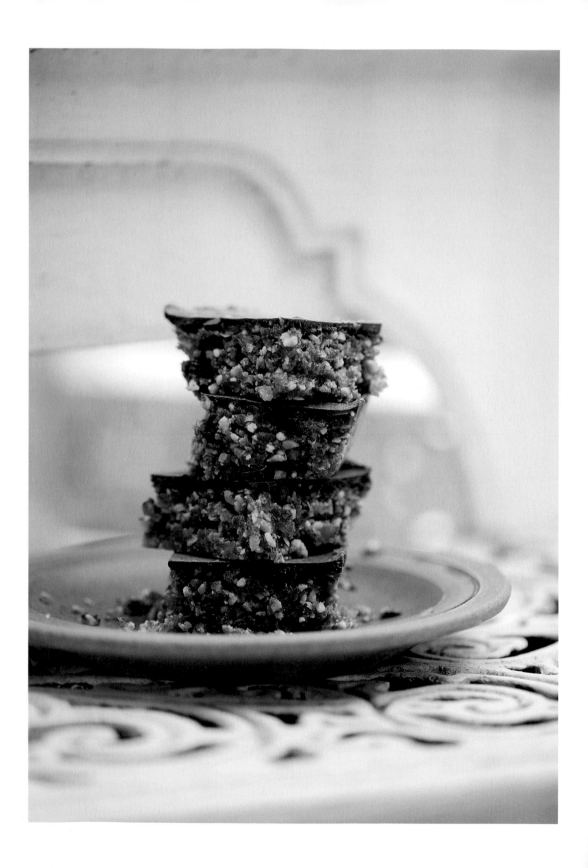

QUINOA, HAZELNUT & CACAO BARS

Another favorite from this book. These slip down too easily, which can be a little dangerous; and half of them can end up disappearing before you've even shared them around! The base layer is amazing: nicely but not sickly sweet and it has such a wonderful array of flavors and textures (I especially love the chewy bites of dried apricots). The chocolate on top adds an indulgent touch, finishing the bars off perfectly.

Makes 20

FOR THE BASE

1 cup plus 2 tablespoons hazelnuts (about
    5½ ounces)

12 medjool dates, pitted

¼ cup almond butter

2 tablespoons tahini

5 tablespoons coconut oil

⅔ cup puffed quinoa

⅓ cup sesame seeds

6 tablespoons raisins

generous 1 cup dried apricots (preferably
    unsulphured), finely chopped

FOR THE CHOCOLATE LAYER

7 ounces cacao butter

5 tablespoons raw cacao powder

6 tablespoons maple syrup

pinch of salt

Preheat the oven to 400°F. Line a rimmed 12 x 8-inch baking sheet with parchment paper.

Roast the hazelnuts on another baking sheet for 10 minutes, then remove from the oven and let cool.

Tip the hazelnuts into a food processor and pulse until broken down into chunks. Put into a large mixing bowl.

Now put the dates into the food processor with the almond butter, tahini and coconut oil. Blend for a minute or so until a smooth paste forms, then add to the hazelnuts in the large mixing bowl. Add all the other base ingredients to the bowl and mix together until completely combined.

Press the mixture into the prepared baking sheet, making sure it is even and quite firmly packed. Place in the fridge to set.

Meanwhile, make the chocolate layer. Combine the cacao butter, cacao powder, maple syrup and salt in a saucepan and place over a really gentle heat until they have melted together; don't let them come to a boil.

Remove the base layer from the fridge and pour the chocolate over the top, then return to the fridge for another 1½ hours to let the chocolate layer set.

Cut into 20 bars to serve. Store any leftovers in the fridge.

PISTACHIO & ORANGE TRUFFLE BITES

The best postdinner treat to serve with tea and coffee. They're gooey and indulgent with an ever-so-slightly chewy texture inside and a crunchy outside. They have smooth chocolatey centers and are rolled in crumbled pistachios to give the perfect finish.

Makes 16–18

6 tablespoons pistachios
12 medjool dates, pitted and chopped
finely grated zest of 1 unwaxed orange,
   plus juice of ½ orange
1 teaspoon coconut oil
3 tablespoons raw cacao powder

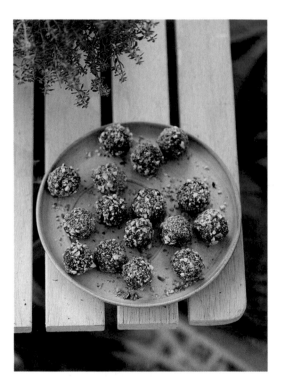

Put the nuts in a food processor and whizz to a crumb-like consistency. Don't worry if they're not all the same size; they're for the truffle coating, so different-size crumbs will add character! When you're happy with the size, tip them into a bowl and set aside.

Throw the dates, orange zest, coconut oil and cacao powder into the processor and whizz it all together. If it gets stuck, use a spatula to push it down toward the blades again and give it another whizz. When it's starting to stick together, squeeze in the orange juice and whizz again until it's a nice sticky consistency that you can roll into balls.

Get a baking sheet ready and wet your hands slightly so that the mixture is easy to roll into balls. Use a teaspoon to get a nice amount together and roll it into a ball. Drop into the nut crumbs and roll it around to coat. Set it on the baking sheet. Repeat to use all the mixture.

Place the baking sheet in the fridge to chill for at least 30 minutes before serving.

MIX IT UP
You can use any nuts you have on hand if you don't want to buy pistachios, but the color of the pistachios makes these look fancy! Or use a mix of chopped pistachios and cashews with pistachio nibs if you want to go all out with eye-catchingly different textures.

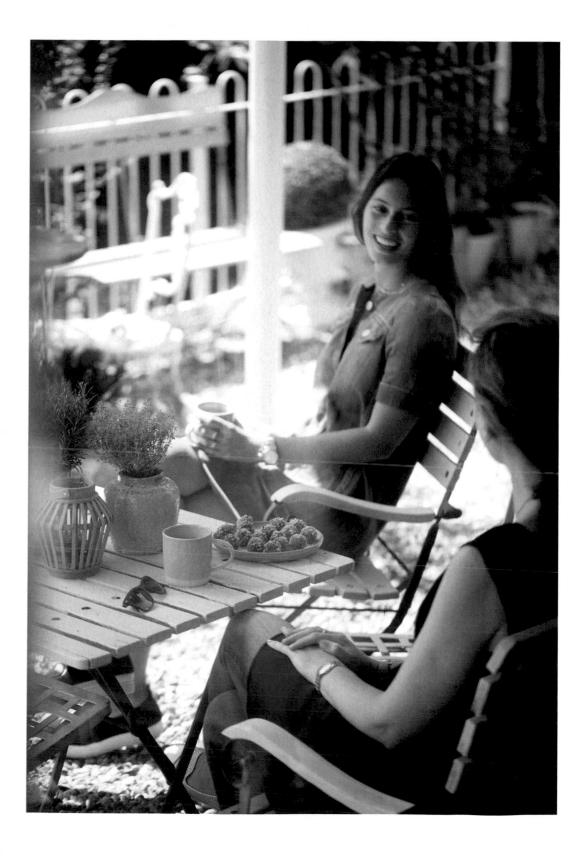

BERRIES WITH CREAMY CHOCOLATE SAUCE & TOASTED NUTS

The perfect dessert for a weekday supper with friends. It just takes fifteen minutes or so to prepare, plus it can't really go wrong, which is a nice feeling when you're a bit tight on time and tired after a long day at work! I like serving this in little bowls, with a bright layer of fresh berries on the bottom and a generous drizzling of warm chocolate sauce and crushed nuts on top. There's nothing fancy about it, but it hits the spot every time.

Serves 4

½ cup pecans

6 tablespoons almonds

3 tablespoons coconut oil

generous ½ cup raw cacao powder

¼ cup plus 2 tablespoons maple syrup

1 tablespoon almond butter, or any other nut butter

scant ¼ cup plant-based milk (I used almond milk)

14 ounces berries (I used blueberries and raspberries, but any fruit works)

Preheat the oven to 400°F.

Place the pecans and almonds on a baking sheet and bake for about 10 minutes, or until crunchy. Set aside to cool.

Heat the coconut oil, cacao powder, maple syrup and almond butter in a saucepan over a gentle heat for a few minutes until it has all melted. Remove from the heat and whisk in the milk to make a smooth sauce.

Roughly chop the nuts, then assemble the dessert. Tumble the berries into 4 bowls, pour over the chocolate sauce, then sprinkle with the chopped nuts. What a treat!

PAN TO PLATE

15 minutes

CLEVER COOKING

This is a great way to use up any leftovers in the house. All fruit works perfectly in this recipe, from grapes to blackberries, strawberries . . . or indeed any fruit you have in the fridge!

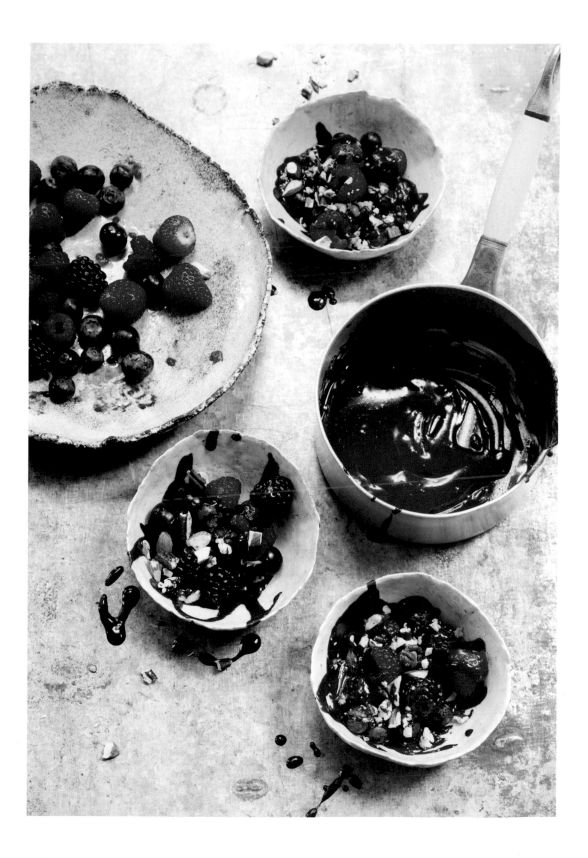

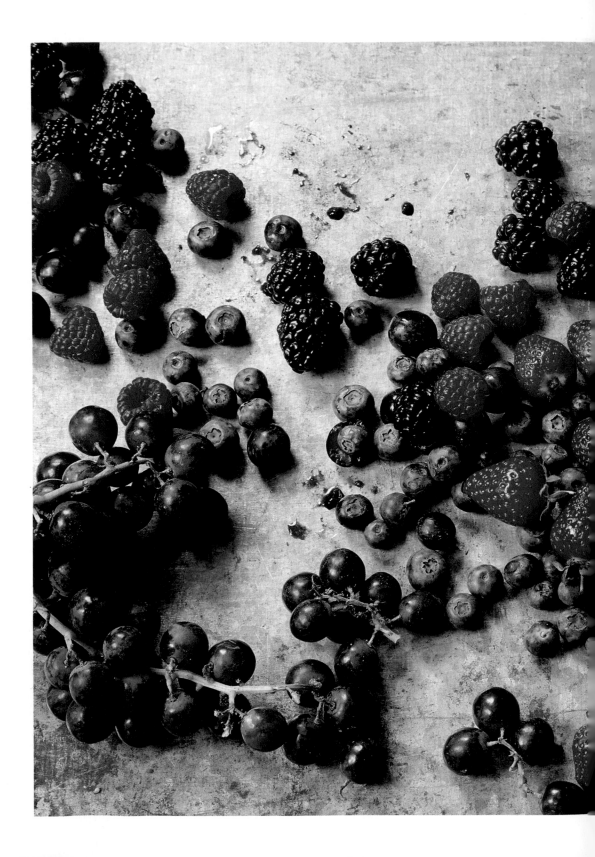

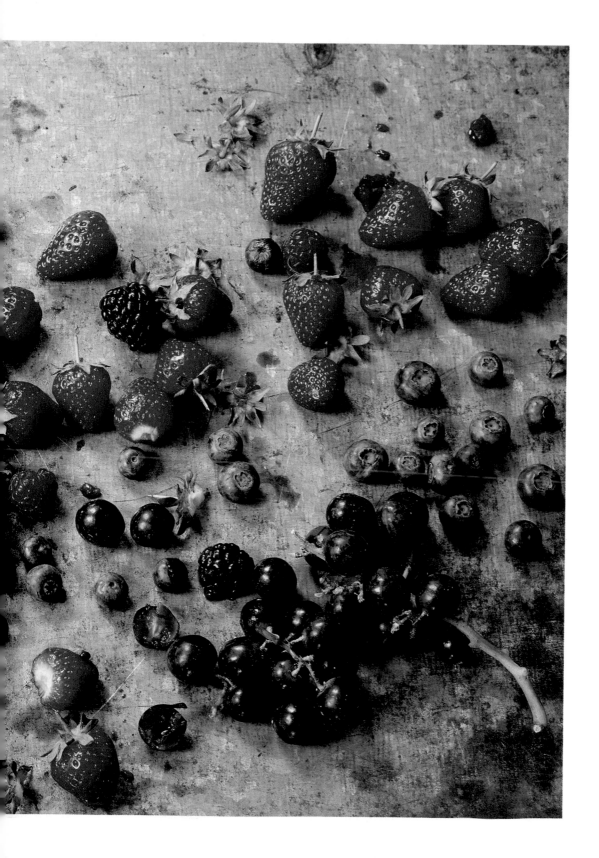

PEACH & COCONUT TART

*This is utter heaven. It's just made to share with friends on a warm summer's day,
so you can sit outside and enjoy every bite. It's also a great recipe for those of you who
don't like overly sweet desserts, but it's still bursting with flavor. I love serving this
slightly warm, with generous scoops of coconut ice cream.*

Makes 1 large tart / Serves 12

6 peaches
7 tablespoons coconut oil
4 tablespoons maple syrup
ground cinnamon
2 tablespoons chia seeds
¾ cup plus 1 tablespoon buckwheat flour
2 cups almond meal
1 tablespoon vanilla powder
¼ cup coconut sugar
¾ cup unsweetened shredded coconut
3 tablespoons coconut chips

Preheat the oven to 400°F. Have a 10 x 11-inch baking dish ready.

Halve and pit the peaches, then slice them. Heat 1 tablespoon of the coconut oil and 1 tablespoon of the maple syrup in a pan and add the peach slices and a sprinkling of cinnamon. Cook for 10 minutes, or until the fruit begins to soften but still holds its shape.

In a small bowl, mix the chia seeds with 6 tablespoons water. Leave for 20 minutes until the seeds expand and form a gel.

Pour the flour, almond meal, vanilla, coconut sugar and remaining 6 tablespoons coconut oil and 3 tablespoons maple syrup into a food processor and blitz until everything has mixed together.

Remove ½ cup of the mix, stir it with the shredded coconut in a bowl and set aside.

Once the chia seeds have soaked up the water, add this to the remaining mixture in the food processor and mix again.

Cut out a sheet of parchment paper to fit the baking dish. Remove the mixture from the food processor and roll it out onto the parchment with a rolling pin, until it is 1 inch thick and covers the parchment completely.

Lift the rolled-out mixture on its parchment base into the dish, then bake for 10 minutes. Remove from the oven and let cool for 5 minutes before scattering half the cooked peaches over the top, squashing down slightly with the back of a wooden spoon. Sprinkle the coconut mixture on top and bake for 20 minutes.

Remove from the oven, add the other half of the peaches, sprinkle with the coconut chips and bake for a final 12 minutes.

Remove from the oven and let cool for about 20 minutes. Then slice, serve and enjoy. Store in an airtight container in the fridge to avoid it going soft.

MIX IT UP
Try serving the Melting Middle Sauce from the Sticky Toffee Pudding (page 270) with this; they taste incredible together!

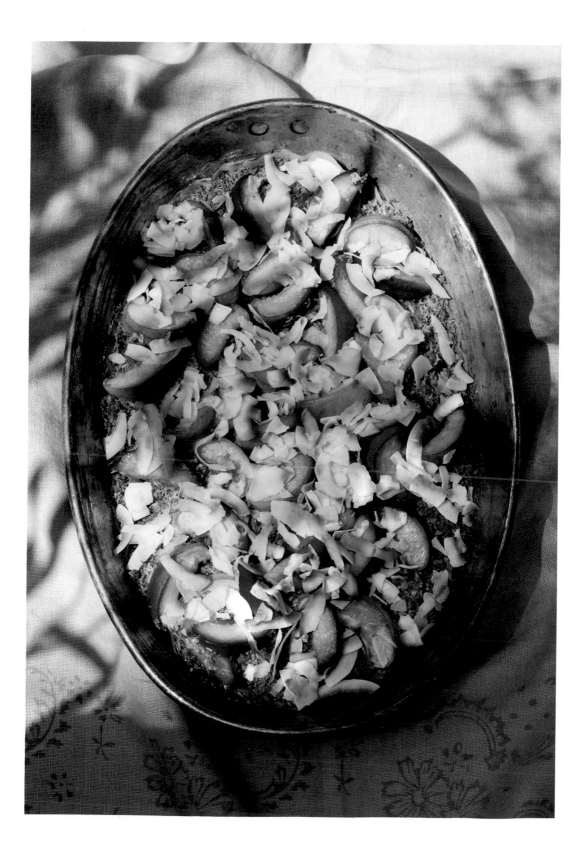

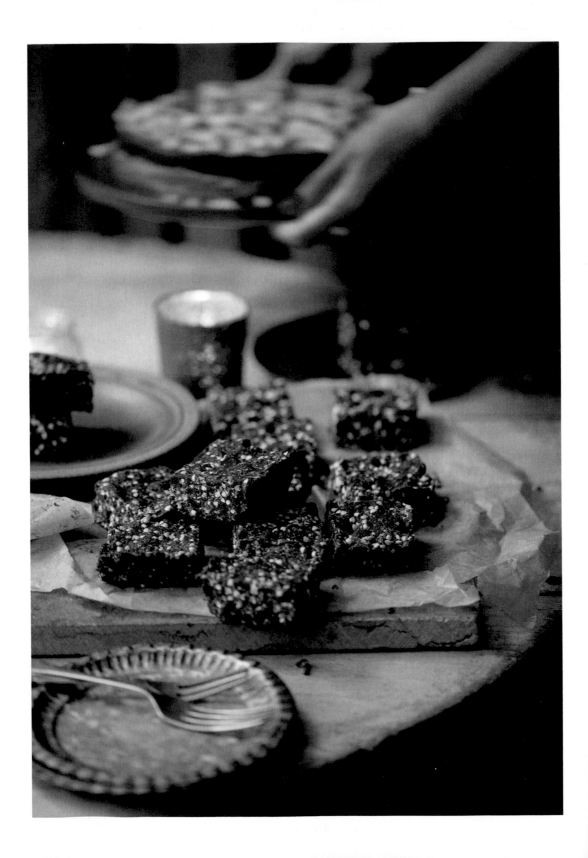

ALMOND BUTTER ROCKY ROADS

It's hard to describe how much I love these. I could happily eat an entire sheet in one sitting . . . and have done so too many times! Each square is wonderfully gooey and chocolatey, with sweet raisins and crunchy toasted buckwheat bites adding extra texture and substance. All I can say is that you just have to go and make them; I promise you'll adore them, too. You can also make them nut-free, with just a couple of tweaks.

Makes 15

scant 1 cup buckwheat groats
3½ ounces cacao butter
2½ cups rolled oats
1 cup pecans (or pumpkin seeds, if you prefer)
11 ounces medjool dates, pitted
2 heaping tablespoons almond butter (or tahini, if you prefer)
5 tablespoons maple syrup
5 tablespoons raw cacao powder
pinch of sea salt
⅓ cup raisins

Preheat the oven to 400°F. Pour the buckwheat groats evenly onto a rimmed baking sheet and bake for 10 minutes, giving the pan a shake halfway through so they all get a bit of color.

Meanwhile, gently heat the cacao butter in a saucepan until melted.

Pour the oats and pecans into a food processor and blitz until they're fully ground down. Add the dates, almond butter, maple syrup, cacao powder, melted cacao butter and salt. Blitz together to form a really smooth and sticky consistency.

Pour the mixture into a large bowl with the raisins and toasted buckwheat and mix well.

Line an 8-inch square brownie pan with parchment, pour in the mixture and smooth it down with a spatula. The mix can be pretty sticky, so make sure you press it well into all the corners. Freeze for about 1 hour, then slice into 15 pieces to serve.

PB&J CAKE

So chocolatey and delicious. Using a mix of dates, banana, peanut butter and coconut oil makes the cake really gooey and fudgy, which is amazing . . . though it's pretty rich. The icing is pretty special, too. I use two layers of goodness to ice it: one mix of peanut butter, maple and vanilla icing and another of smashed raspberries with coconut sugar; you can only imagine how good they taste together, especially with the rich chocolate cake. It's the perfect treat for any celebratory meal, or your reward after a weekend baking session.

Serves 8–10

FOR THE CAKE

1 tablespoon coconut oil, plus more
   for the pans
1¾ cups plus 2 tablespoons rolled oats
1½ cups almond meal
¾ cup plus 2 tablespoons brown rice milk
2 avocados, peeled and pitted

10 medjool dates, pitted
½ cup plus 2 tablespoons raw cacao powder
½ cup maple syrup
5 tablespoons coconut sugar
5 tablespoons peanut butter
¼ cup chia seeds
1 small overripe banana (3 ounces with skin
   on), mashed
pinch of salt

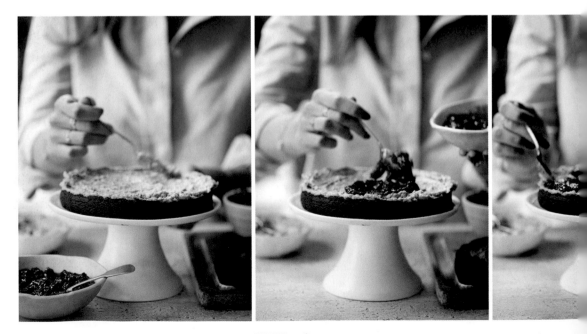

FOR THE ICING

¾ cup cashews, soaked for 2–4 hours and drained

3 tablespoons maple syrup

3 tablespoons peanut butter

½ tablespoon coconut oil

½ tablespoon coconut sugar

1 teaspoon vanilla powder

FOR THE RASPBERRY LAYER

2 cups raspberries, plus more to serve

2 tablespoons coconut sugar, plus more to serve

Preheat the oven to 400°F. Oil two 8- or 9-inch cake pans with coconut oil.

Tip the oats into a food processor and blend until a flour forms. Add all the other ingredients (not forgetting the 1 tablespoon of coconut oil) and blend until a thick, chocolatey mix forms. Divide the batter between the prepared pans.

Bake for about 50 minutes, until a knife poked in comes out clean. Let the cakes cool in the pans (they'll finish setting while they cool).

Meanwhile, make the icing. Tip the drained cashews into a blender. Add all the other ingredients with ¼ cup water. Blitz, then scrape out into a bowl and let it sit in the fridge for 10 minutes or so to firm up.

For the raspberry layer, mash the raspberries on a plate, stirring in the coconut sugar.

Turn the cakes out of the pans and place the least attractive layer flat side up on a cake plate. Spread with half the icing, then top with half the mashed raspberries. Place the other layer on top, flat sides together, and do the same again. Arrange some raspberries over the top. I like to sprinkle a little extra coconut sugar on top as a final flourish, as it looks beautiful.

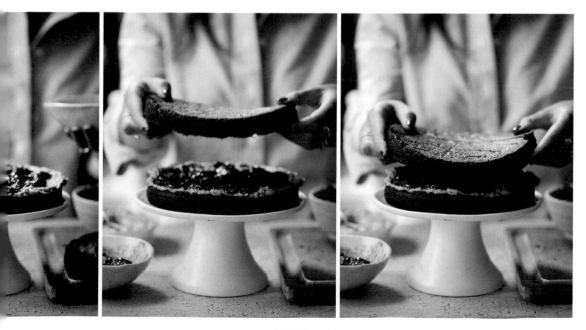

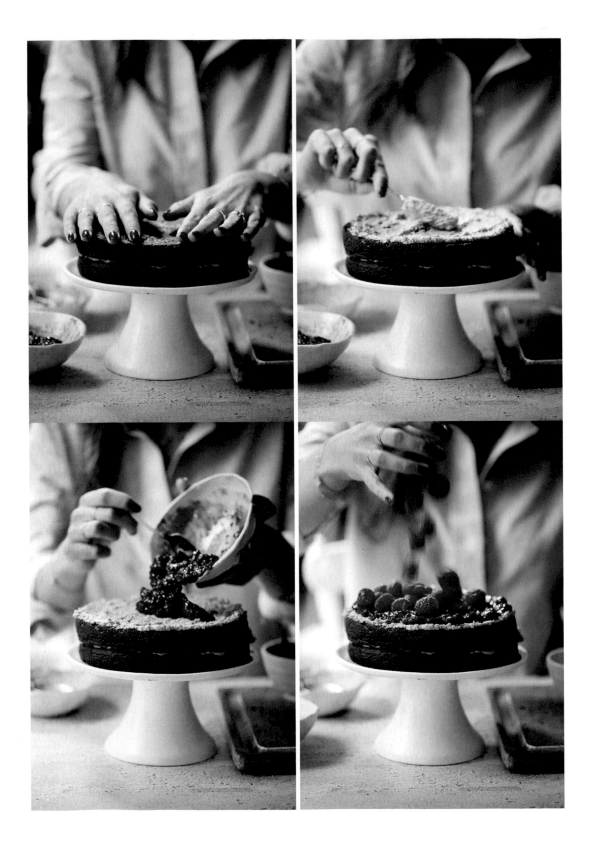

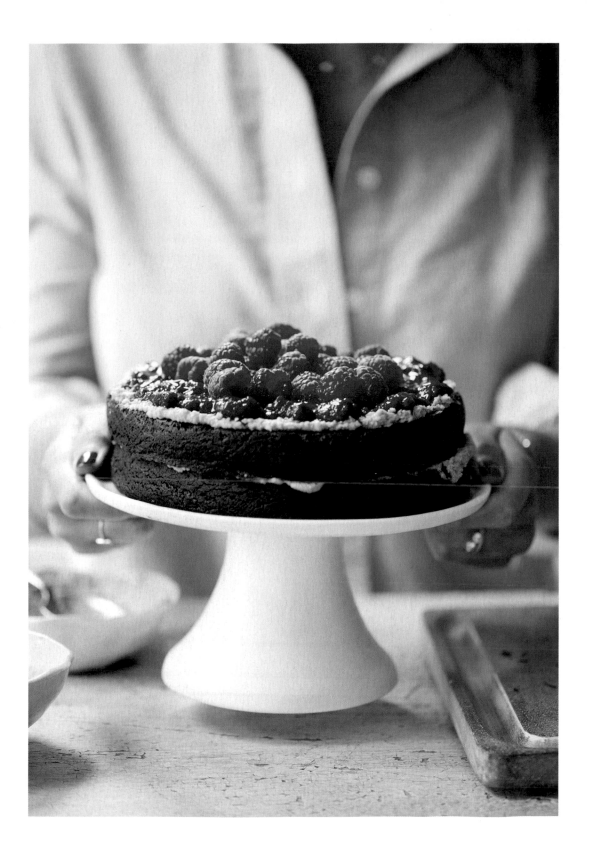

CHOCOLATE-ORANGE TART

Anything chocolate-orange-focused is always such a winner; it's a classic combination of flavors that everyone seems to love. This creamy tart is no exception. The almond and orange base has subtle hints of cacao, coconut and maple, which perfectly complement the sweet, creamy middle. The tart is then finished off with a beautiful scattering of orange zest and salt, which heightens the flavors and makes it look perfect.

Serves 10–12

FOR THE BASE

2 tablespoons coconut oil, plus more
   for the pan
1 cup almonds
2 tablespoons raw cacao powder
5 ounces medjool dates, pitted
finely grated zest of 1 unwaxed orange,
   plus juice of ½ orange
pinch of salt
1 tablespoon maple syrup

FOR THE MIDDLE LAYER

2 avocados
4 heaping tablespoons raw cacao powder
¼ cup date syrup
2 tablespoons coconut oil
2 tablespoons honey
2 tablespoons peanut or almond butter
finely grated zest and juice of
   2 unwaxed oranges
pinch of salt

TO DECORATE

finely grated zest of ½ unwaxed orange
pinch of flaky sea salt

Oil an 8-inch springform pan with coconut oil, or line it with parchment paper.

Make the base. Start by blitzing the almonds in a food processor until they form a chunky flour, then add all the other ingredients (not forgetting the 2 tablespoons of coconut oil) and blend until a sticky mixture forms. Use a spatula to firmly press the mixture down into the prepared pan. Place in the freezer for 30 minutes to set the tart base.

Meanwhile, make the middle layer. Scoop the avocado flesh into a food processor. Add the other ingredients and blend until a smooth, creamy, mousse-like mixture forms.

Pour it over the base, then return to the freezer for 1 hour to set. Take it out about 15 minutes before serving.

Grate the orange zest over the top and sprinkle with a few flakes of sea salt.

Store any leftovers in the freezer.

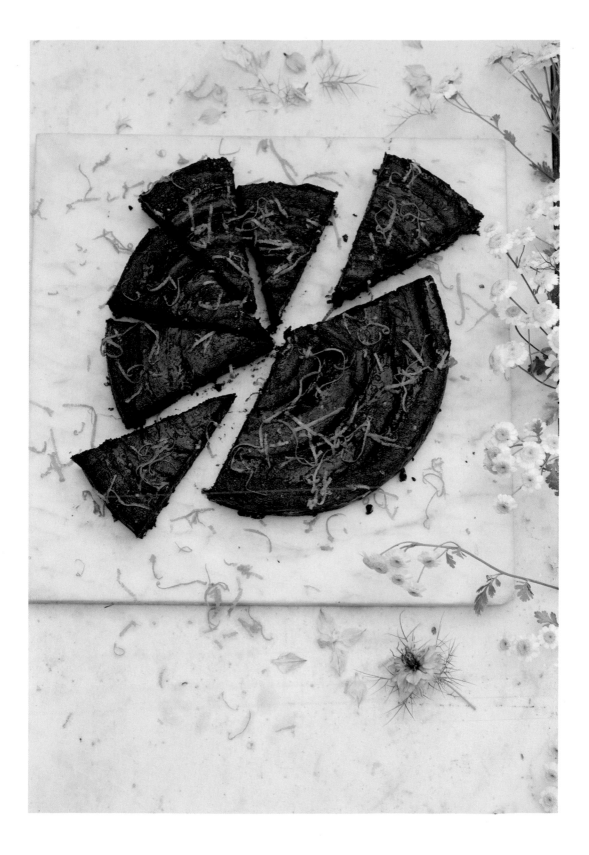

CHOCOLATE PEANUT BUTTER PIE

Who doesn't love the sound of this?! It is real indulgence: sweet, rich, nutty and oh so delicious. It's also pretty filling, so you may want to cut your guests relatively small slices to start with and serve it alongside some dollops of coconut yogurt to lighten it up. My ultimate treat. I hope it will be yours, too!

Serves 12

FOR THE CHOCOLATE LAYER

½ cup plus 1 tablespoon coconut oil, plus more for the pan

1 cup plus 2 tablespoons raw cacao powder

1½ tablespoons cacao butter

1 teaspoon vanilla powder

¼ cup peanut butter

3 tablespoons honey

5 tablespoons coconut sugar

pinch of salt

FOR THE BASE

2½ cups rolled oats

3 tablespoons coconut oil

2 tablespoons peanut butter

1½ tablespoons honey

1 teaspoon vanilla powder

pinch of salt

FOR THE MIDDLE LAYER AND TOPPING

generous ½ cup peanut butter

1–2 tablespoons unsalted raw peanuts, roughly chopped

Oil an 8-inch springform pan with coconut oil, or line it with parchment paper.

Make the chocolate layer first. Simply place all the ingredients into a saucepan over a low heat and gently stir until melted and mixed together. Set aside to cool and thicken.

Meanwhile, make the base. Whizz the oats in a food processor to a flour, then add all the other ingredients, with 2 tablespoons water and 2 tablespoons of the chocolate layer mix. Blend until a sticky mix forms. Press into the prepared pan so it's tightly packed, then place in the freezer for 10–15 minutes to firm up.

For the middle layer, spread the peanut butter evenly over the base, then freeze for 10 minutes to set.

Finally, pour the chocolate layer over and sprinkle with the peanuts. Let it set in the fridge for 30 minutes before serving. Be patient! It really does need the setting time.

Store any leftovers in the fridge or freezer.

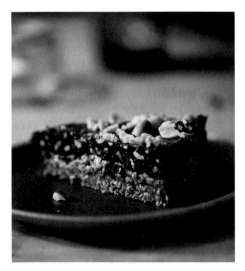

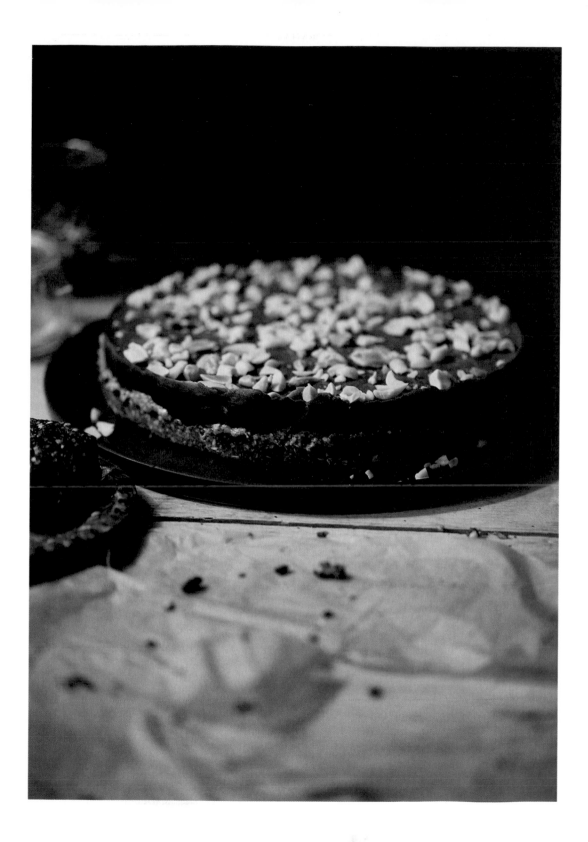

STICKY TOFFEE PUDDING

Growing up, sticky toffee pudding was my and my siblings' favorite dessert. We were all obsessed with it and would ask for it all the time . . . we even used to have it on Christmas Day. I'm sure part of the reason I love it so much is that it's a celebration of sweet, sticky dates and—as lots of you know—I adore dates, so any dessert where they're the focus is always a winner in my book! This is a really indulgent way to end a meal, and absolutely nothing about it looks or tastes healthy, so it's ideal if you've got a few skeptical friends coming over and you need a real treat to serve them. It is great served with coconut yogurt or coconut ice cream, which adds a lovely refreshing touch.

Serves 8

FOR THE MELTING MIDDLE SAUCE

7 ounces medjool dates, pitted

3 tablespoons coconut oil

2 tablespoons maple syrup

2 tablespoons coconut sugar

pinch of salt

FOR THE PUDDING

7 ounces medjool dates, pitted

2 tablespoons flaxseeds

1 cup plus 5 tablespoons almond meal

½ cup cornmeal

2 tablespoons coconut sugar

2 tablespoons maple syrup

2 tablespoons date syrup

1 teaspoon vanilla powder

pinch of salt

Start with the sauce. Place the dates in a pan with the coconut oil over low heat. Allow them to melt and warm together for about 5 minutes, until the dates are nice and soft. Pour this into a blender with the maple syrup, coconut sugar and salt, then pour in 1 cup water. Blend until a deliciously smooth, thick sauce forms.

For the pudding, put the dates in a saucepan with 1 cup water. Cook over low heat until a sticky paste forms, then set aside. In a bowl, soak the flaxseeds with ¼ cup water for 10 minutes, so it starts to thicken. Mix the date paste and flaxseeds with all the other ingredients in a large mixing bowl.

Line a 1-quart mixing bowl with parchment paper. Spoon 5 tablespoons of the sauce into the bowl, then spoon the pudding mixture on top. Tie parchment over the bowl with string to secure. Put it in a wide pan and fill the pan with boiling water to come halfway up the bowl. Cover, place over medium heat and bring to a simmer. Simmer for 1½ hours. Check on the water level every 30 minutes to be sure it hasn't evaporated, which might burn the pudding or crack the bowl.

Place a serving plate on top of the bowl and flip to unmold the pudding. Leave it there for about 10 minutes while you reheat the sauce for drizzling over the top!

CLEVER COOKING

I often make extra sauce, as I can never get enough of it with this pudding!

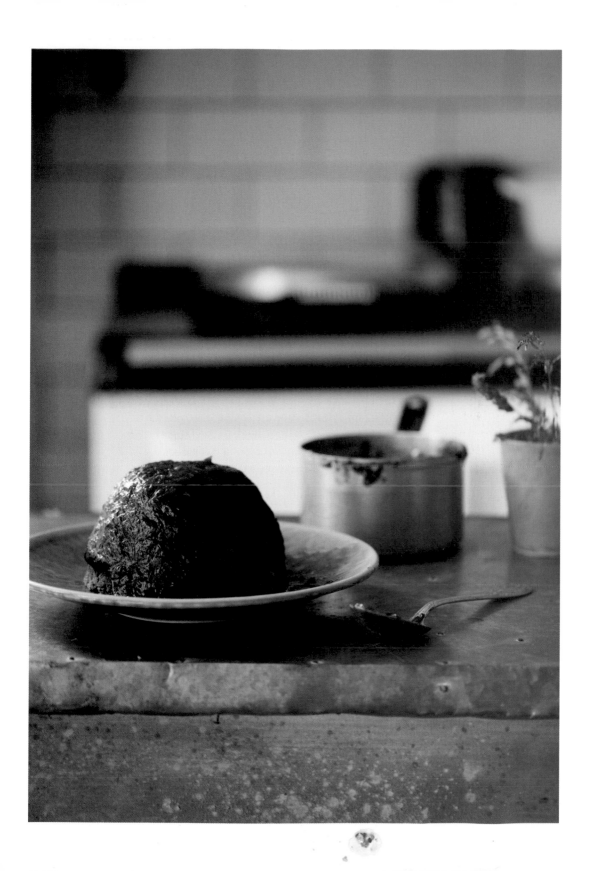

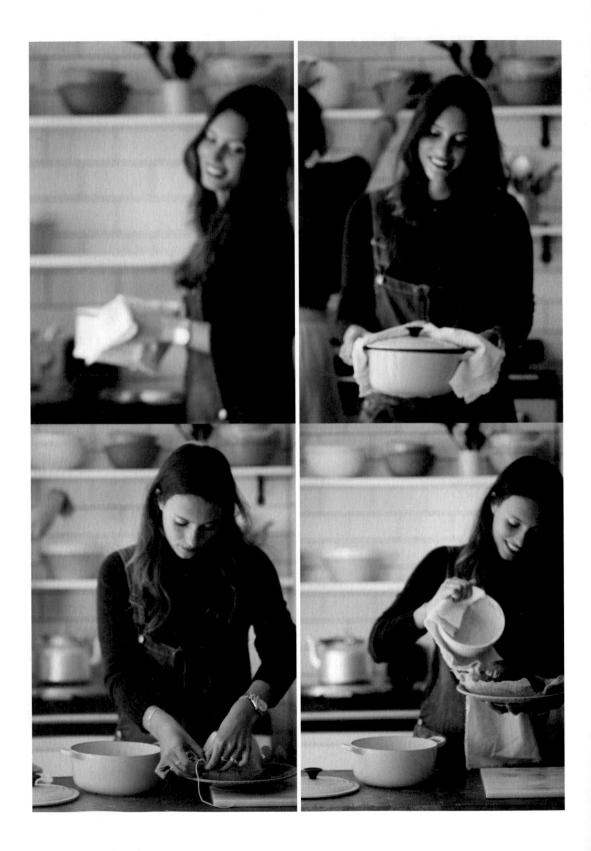

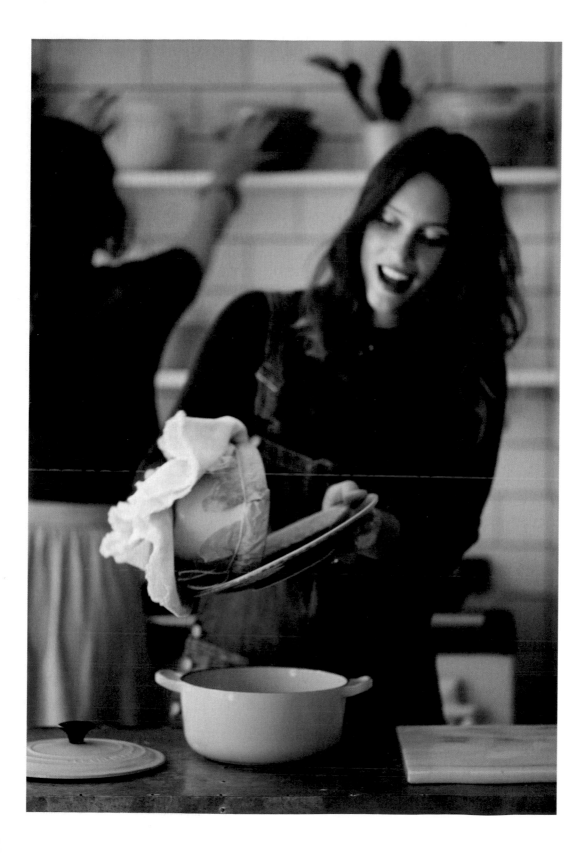

ORANGE & POLENTA CAKE

Definitely the Deliciously Ella office's favorite cake. Every time this has been made it seems to get devoured within minutes and we can't wait for it to be recipe tested again! It's lighter than the PB&J Cake (page 262), with lovely hints of almond and orange. My favorite part is the orange and coconut sugar glaze, which is not only incredibly flavorful, but also very beautiful. This works perfectly served at room temperature, but it's also amazing served straight out of the oven with some coconut or cashew ice cream for a warming treat in the winter, or even on a cool summer evening.

Serves 12

FOR THE CAKE

3 tablespoons coconut oil, plus more
    for the pan (optional)
2½ tablespoons chia seeds
1½ teaspoons apple cider vinegar
¾ cup almond milk
¾ cup maple syrup
2 teaspoons vanilla powder
2 cups fine polenta
3 cups almond meal
2 tablespoons plus 1 teaspoon arrowroot
    powder
finely grated zest of ½ unwaxed lemon
finely grated zest and juice of
    1 unwaxed orange
pinch of salt

FOR THE GLAZE

finely grated zest and juice of
    2 unwaxed oranges
finely grated zest of 1 unwaxed lemon
¼ cup coconut sugar

Preheat the oven to 380°F. Oil an 8-inch round cake pan with coconut oil, or line it with parchment paper.

Spoon the chia seeds into a cup, pour in 6 tablespoons water and set aside for 20 minutes, until a gel forms.

Gently heat the 3 tablespoons of coconut oil until it melts.

In a large mixing bowl, combine all the cake ingredients, including the chia mixture and coconut oil. Stir until combined and smooth.

Spoon into the prepared pan and bake for 45–50 minutes, until golden brown and a knife poked into the middle comes out clean.

Meanwhile, make the glaze. Gently heat the orange zest and juice, lemon zest and coconut sugar in a saucepan until the sugar dissolves and a thin syrup forms.

Let the cake cool for 20 minutes in the pan on a cooling rack. Remove from the pan, then evenly drizzle the syrup and zest before serving.

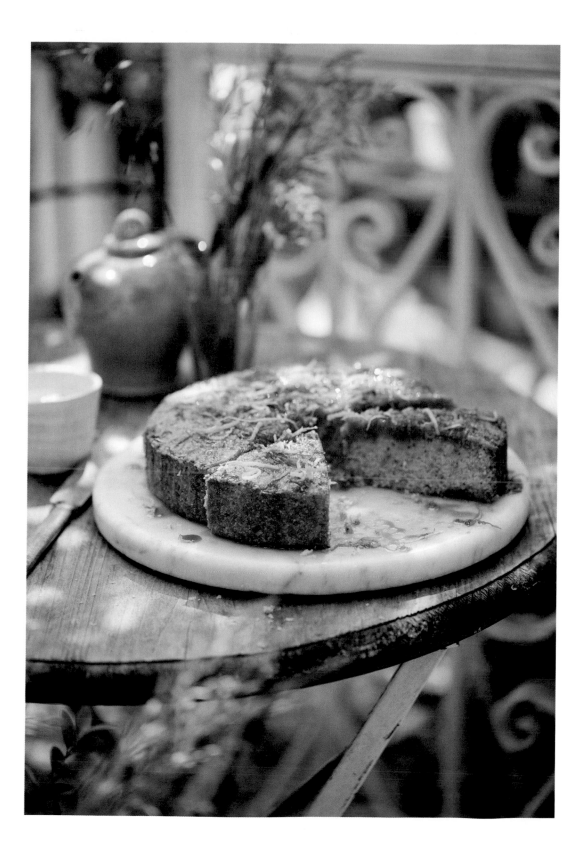

ICE CREAM SUNDAES

This is a pretty exciting dessert, filled with chewy bites of hazelnut brownie, soft scoops of banana ice cream infused with chunks of dates and your favorite nut butter, creamy chocolate sauce and then a sprinkling of toasted hazelnuts, coconut chips and a handful of sweet berries. YUM! It's a little fussy to make as there are a few different elements to it, but it's so worth doing every now and again when you want something that feels like a wonderful treat.

Serves 4

FOR THE HAZELNUT BROWNIE BITES
½ cup plus 1 tablespoon roasted hazelnuts
7 ounces medjool dates, pitted
2 tablespoons raw cacao powder

FOR THE CHOCOLATE SAUCE
generous ½ cup raw cacao powder
6 tablespoons date syrup
2 tablespoons coconut oil
3 tablespoons coconut milk

FOR THE ICE CREAM
8 very ripe bananas, thinly sliced and frozen
    for at least 4 hours
¼ cup crunchy nut butter (peanut, almond
    and cashew are all great)
12 medjool dates, pitted and
    roughly chopped

TO SERVE
berries
toasted hazelnuts (optional)
coconut chips (optional)

Make the brownie bites. Place the hazelnuts in a food processor and blitz until they're crushed, then add the dates and cacao and blend until a sticky mixture forms. Scrape the mixture out, press it into a rimmed baking sheet, cover and leave in the fridge until you need it.

Once you're ready for your sundaes, make the chocolate sauce. Melt the cacao powder, date syrup and coconut oil together in saucepan, then whisk in the coconut milk. Set aside to cool.

Make the ice cream. Take the bananas out of the freezer and let them thaw for a few minutes. Meanwhile, chop the brownie mix into bite-size chunks.

Place the bananas in a food processor and blend for a minute or so, until totally smooth and resembling soft-serve ice cream. Add the nut butter and blend for another few seconds. Stir in the dates (don't blend them in; you want them to be chunky).

Put a few brownie bites and berries at the bottom of 4 serving glasses or bowls, then add a scoop or two of ice cream, more brownie bites, chocolate sauce and toasted hazelnuts or coconut chips, if you like.

Serve straightaway so the ice cream doesn't melt!

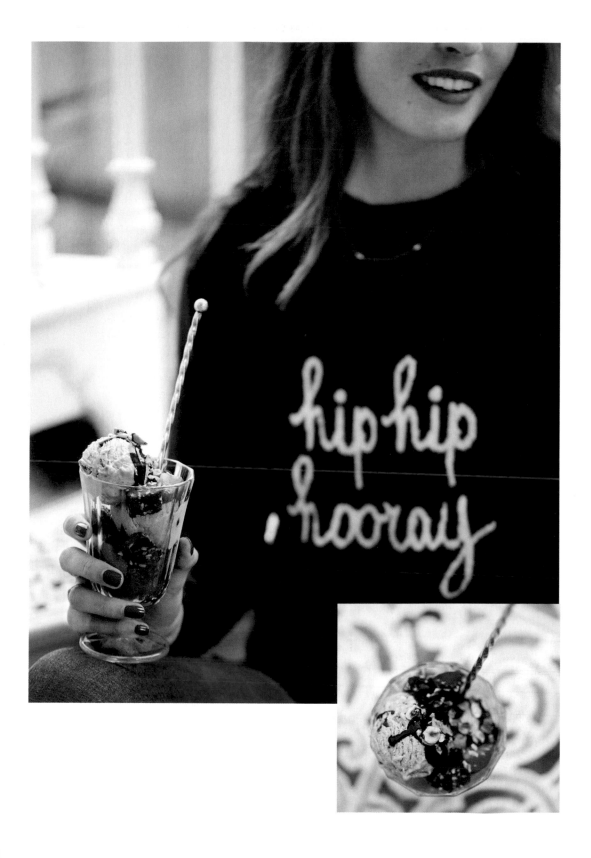

RECIPE INDEX

INDEX

THANK YOU

Every time I write a book I feel the list of people I want to thank gets longer and longer, as more incredible people enter my life and support Deliciously Ella!

It goes without saying that my readers get the biggest thank-you. You've made my entire career possible and I'll forever be grateful for your daily support and enthusiasm for what I do. It inspires me so much and it's the reason that I continue to share recipes and ideas with the world. Together we've created a really special community, and I'm incredibly proud of the journey that we're sharing.

To my husband, Matthew, it's hard to find the right words to thank you for everything you do every day. The unending kindness and encouragement you show me is unbelievable: not only have you become my sounding board for every idea, you also help me nurture and grow the idea and inspire me to push myself in everything I do. You've motivated me to aim higher, believe in myself more and—most important— be the best and kindest person I can be, for which I am forever grateful.

Our team at Deliciously Ella and the delis also deserve a huge thank-you. Serena, Jess and Laura Kate are my daily support at Deliciously Ella and allow me to share more with you. I can't thank them enough for their hard work, laughter, creativity and positive energy, as well as their amazing ability to eat as much as I do and recipe test every day! Our team at the delis is building an amazing company with Matthew and me, which allows us to share my philosophy with so many more people, and that makes me so incredibly happy. Isabella, Tom, Dan, Alan, Holly, Betty, Ed and Lorna . . . You're wonderful.

Thank you to Cathryn, Gordy, Siobhan, Chekka and everyone else at WME that supports Deliciously Ella. Your advice and guidance are invaluable and there's no way that I could have grown Deliciously Ella into what it is now without your encouragement and guidance.

Liz, Louise, Vickie and the team at Yellow Kite and Hodder, thank you all so much for believing in what I'm doing. It means the world to me to have such a dedicated publisher that shares my vision and really believes in the message I want to share with you all. Working together is always an incredibly collaborative, creative process and that really makes the book so special.

It's also thanks to Miranda, Clare, Rosie, Ellie, Polly and Lucy that the books look and feel so beautiful. Your hard work and imagination have brought my vision to life in a way that's so much better than I could have imagined. Thanks to you the recipes look stunning and I hope will inspire more people to get cooking! Thank you for helping me share this with the world in the best possible way.

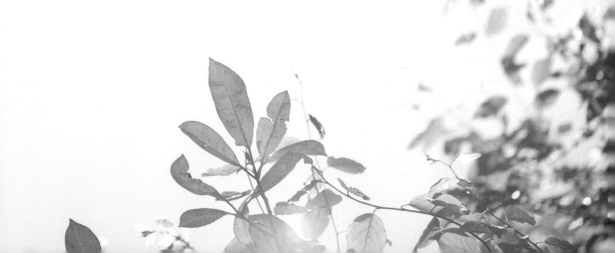

Scribner
An Imprint of Simon & Schuster, Inc.
1230 Avenue of the Americas
New York, NY 10020

First Scribner hardcover edition October 2017

SCRIBNER and design are registered trademarks of The Gale Group, Inc., used under license by Simon & Schuster, Inc., the publisher of this work.

For information about special discounts for bulk purchases, please contact Simon & Schuster Special Sales at 1-866-506-1949 or business@simonandschuster.com.

The Simon & Schuster Speakers Bureau can bring authors to your live event. For more information or to book an event, contact the Simon & Schuster Speakers Bureau at 1-866-248-3049 or visit our website at www.simonspeakers.com.

Interior design by Miranda Harvey

Endpapers © Shutterstock

Manufactured in the United States of America

10 9 8 7 6 5 4 3 2 1

Library of Congress Cataloging-in-Publication Data is available.

ISBN 978-1-5011-7427-8
ISBN 978-1-5011-7428-5 (ebook)

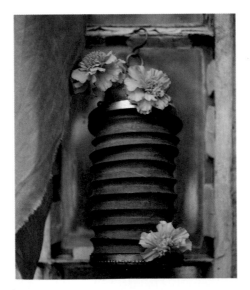